Increasing IVF Success with Acupuncture

of related interest

Eight Extraordinary Channels – Qi Jing Ba Mai
A Handbook for Clinical Practice and Nei Dan Inner Meditation
Dr David Twicken DOM, LAc
ISBN 978 1 84819 148 8
eISBN 978 0 85701 137 4

The Compleat Acupuncturist
A Guide to Constitutional and Conditional Pulse Diagnosis
Peter Eckman
Foreword by William Morris
ISBN 978 1 84819 198 3
eISBN 978 0 85701 152 7

Common Laboratory Tests Used by TCM Practitioners
When to Refer Patients for Lab Tests and How to Read and Interpret the Results
Partha Banerjee MD and Christina Captain
ISBN 978 1 84819 205 8
eISBN 978 0 85701 164 0

Increasing IVF Success with Acupuncture

An Integrated Approach

NICK DALTON-BREWER, MSc

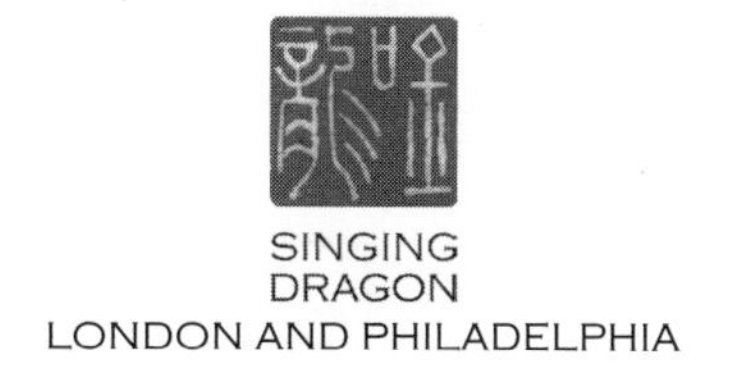

SINGING
DRAGON
LONDON AND PHILADELPHIA

First published in 2014
by Singing Dragon
an imprint of Jessica Kingsley Publishers
73 Collier Street
London N1 9BE, UK
and
400 Market Street, Suite 400
Philadelphia, PA 19106, USA

www.singingdragon.com

Library of Congress Cataloging in Publication Data
Dalton-Brewer, Nick, author.
Increasing IVF success with acupuncture : an integrated approach / Nick Dalton-Brewer.
p. ; cm.
Increasing in vitro fertilization success with acupuncture
Includes bibliographical references and index.
ISBN 978-1-84819-218-8 (alk. paper)
I. Title. II. Title: Increasing in vitro fertilization success with acupuncture.
[DNLM: 1. Reproductive Techniques, Assisted. 2. Acupuncture Therapy. 3. Integrative Medicine. 4.
Medicine, Chinese Traditional. WQ 208]
RG135
618.1'780599--dc23
2014007991

British Library Cataloguing in Publication Data
A CIP catalogue record for this book is available from the British Library

ISBN 978 1 84819 218 8
eISBN 978 0 85701 165 7

Printed and bound in Great Britain

CONTENTS

1

Acupuncture

An Introduction

This book is written to explore factors implicated in female fertility and its treatment. Although it mainly considers how female fertility is influenced, male fertility is also raised, and particularly the recent rapid decline in sperm parameters. If you are interested in artificial reproduction, as a traditional Chinese medicine practitioner, a student, a patient, or you simply have an interest in reproduction and health, then this book is for you.

Sex selection, artificial reproduction, the exclusion of hereditable diseases: in this century, not only are these possible, they are available. The world is changing far faster than we know or can appreciate. Less than 150 years ago, the telephone was invented, the long-lasting light bulb was made, the first car was built by Daimler. Now we are looking at some of the deepest interrelationships in life. Who would have thought it? Now human cloning is a very real possibility and it will more likely not be restricted by technology but solely by ethics. Silicon may be at an end, and organic computers may be conceived. As we delve deeper and faster, who knows what we will unearth?

Until very recently, the dominant culture was Western, and ideas and information travelled from the West to the East. In the very near future, the dominant economy will be Eastern, and culture will travel from the East to the West.

The difference between cultures is not just based in history, but in the way individuals from the West or the East perceive the world. In the main, people raised in the West are thought to perceive the world objectively, that is context independently, whilst people raised in an Eastern culture perceive the world contextually. On the whole, this difference underpins all aspects in each culture. People from an Eastern culture will tend to think in terms of relationships, whereas for people from a Western culture, objects will stand out more than relationships. For example, when shown groups of words, people raised in a Western culture tend to group them as objects, semantically (e.g. adult and child), whereas people from East Asia tend to group them thematically (e.g. woman and baby). The perception is not simply skin deep; entirely different brain structures are used.[1]

Medicine is the art and science of healing, a reflection of culture. The type of medicine that is available, that is practised, that is used to treat and used to develop treatments is cultural in origin. In the art of medicine, however, the patient narrative is essential; traditional Chinese medicine is a context-driven system, the yin perhaps to Western conventional medicine's object-based yang. It is this difference between the two systems that proffers such opportunities when integrated. There is an awful lot that Western conventional medicine can do which traditional Chinese medicine cannot; and there is an awful lot that traditional Chinese medicine can do that Western conventional medicine cannot. The intersection of these two systems, the integration of them, could prove significantly beneficial for patients.

Traditional Chinese medicine (TCM) practitioners who were brought up in the West, and who trained in TCM in the West, have developed a unique perspective. First, Western people are essentially object based, and the system of medicine learnt by TCM practitioners is derived from China, a context-based culture. Moreover, TCM is a narrative/context-based system of medicine. Second, the system of medicine originates from a time more remote than anything that could possibly be compared to in the West, predating the Bible by at least a thousand years – ancient China is a culture so remote that its origins are lost in the mists of time. As Claude Larre points out, 'The fact is that the way the Chinese express themselves is conveyed to us through means which are very far from our alphabetic languages in the Occident.'[2] To practise this system of medicine, the Western TCM practitioner has to understand another culture originating from another time and still practised in the modern world, and to be able to carry both cultural perspectives equally. This combination of factors enables a truly unique perspective.

To be able to increase the rate of pregnancy and live birth rate, as research studies have shown, acupuncture must be able to create physiological change. It is now generally accepted that one of the pathways by which acupuncture does this is through the neuroendocrine system. Some few years ago, a friend of mine said, 'There's no point planning a venture when we don't have the technology.' We were talking about the autocrine/paracrine systems, and how acupuncture might modulate these to improve fertility, uterine receptivity and reproductive capacity. Now, more than ever before, with advances in technology, it's possible to evaluate what's going on in those systems and other systems known to influence in vitro fertilisation (IVF) outcome. Since everything is energy, molecular biology is a good place to start when considering different types of energy donors and different types of energy states, especially when thinking about oxidative stress and the antioxidants required to combat it.

Change is the immutable law in the universe. Just as the world is changing, with ideas and knowledge being exchanged at an ever-increasing rate, so are we looking at transitions in medicine. Managing change relies on maintaining balance. Too much change is known to cause illness. It may be that the pace of change is at the heart of the epidemics now facing our civilisation and which are discussed in this book, particularly stress, obesity and the rapid decline in fertility.

Changes in health in Western populations may also be due to endocrinological factors, corrupted by endocrine disrupting compounds (EDCs). The existence of these and other compounds in our food chain may be the ultimate cause of modern epidemics, or may be exacerbating the failing health of populations. Whatever the cause, acquiring an understanding of the hormonal axes involved, molecular co-relationships, and the processes and effects of signalling involved in healthy fertility can be a helpful step when considering treatments for fertility.

Acupuncture

Acupuncture has evolved from the mists of time. Empirical evidence derived from texts, letters, books and compendia written over the centuries by traditional doctors shows analyses of acupuncture techniques and point prescriptions used during clinical practice, outcomes observed, warnings and successes, and theoretical exposition, much like twenty-first-century risk management systems.

During the millennia that it has been used to help people, acupuncture has relied on traditional techniques, skills, and common understanding of a cosmology that is still practised by more people on this world than not. Its very pragmatism has enabled its flexibility, and its efficacy has maintained health for centuries. The current century is seeing a new development in the history of acupuncture and its integration with Western medical techniques and technologies. With this integration, the therapy is evolving.

Molecular medicine, genetics, neuroendocrinology and other rapidly evolving modern medicine systems all represent opportunities to extend human understanding in health and evolution. The acupuncture system, with its unique capacity to deliver physical and emotional change whilst being biochemically inert (virtually) differentiates treatment from pharmaceuticals, which interact with so many physical systems. This differentiation proffers great promise. Treatments with acupuncture can provide a biochemically inert adjunctive therapy working in concert with pharmaceutical therapies or as a stand-alone therapy. In the former case, I am sure you can see the benefit to patients, where treatment regimes burdened by biochemical interactions could be augmented by a biochemically inert therapy. It could even prove beneficial in research.

Is acupuncture a philosophy or a science?

Acupuncture belongs to a group of therapies that comprise TCM, which includes Chinese herbal medicine, massage exercise and nutritional therapy. These therapies rely on the same fundamental system of diagnosis, pathogenic factors and treatment principles – the medical system. At the heart of this system is the understanding that all systems work most effectively where there is balance, that is, homeostasis. In the traditional world, TCM was used to keep someone healthy, hence the old phrase 'It is advisable to sharpen your sword before you go into battle.'

It is quite reasonable to suggest that traditional acupuncture makes use of a scientific method, where science is the systematic method of acquiring knowledge to comprehend the environment, with the use of careful observation, experiment, measurement, mathematics and replication.

Philosophy: love of wisdom; from the Greek *philo* (love), *sophos* (wisdom). The guiding principles of TCM and therefore acupuncture are derived from the culture of Taoism and the writings of Confucius, both of which are very much related to understanding society and consciousness.

When we consider authors such as Teichmann and Evans, where philosophy 'is a study of problems which are ultimate, abstract and very general' and 'concerned with the nature of existence, knowledge, morality, reason and human purpose' or Grayling, where the aim of philosophy is 'to gain insight into questions about knowledge, truth, reason, reality, meaning, mind, and value' we can say that TCM is also philosophical.[3, 4]

From a pragmatic point of view, in traditional times, if a doctor did not heal the patient, the doctor wouldn't get paid. It would therefore behove the doctor to love knowledge and wisdom very much indeed!

Finally, the practice of TCM relies very much on a practical understanding of the traditional Chinese concept of energy, qi (pronounced chee). Chinese philosophers considered qi both tangible and intanglible.[5] A similar concept of energy is found in the West, where the measurement of energy is in reference to the capacity of a system's ability to work.[6] A concept of energy per se is meaningless: 'only change in energy has meaning',[7] and so in Western thought, energy transitions between states. Different types of energy are identifiable, for example, kinetic, electrical or thermal. In TCM terms human physiology is based on transitions of energy and, amongst other attributes, relates to the functions of the organs and pathology.[8] For example, liver functions include the smooth flow of energy and supply of liver blood to the uterus. During times when the liver must work harder, during the menses for instance, these functions may become impaired, and liver energy may stagnate; blood flow may become uneven, and cramping pain may ensue.

Is acupuncture effective?

TCM has been the primary medical system in China and Japan for centuries and is fundamentally integrated with Western conventional medicine (WCM) in the Chinese medical system. Last year, there were probably more than a billion people to whom this question would not have occurred. More likely the question asked would be: 'Was the doctor good?'

Evidence for the effectiveness of acupuncture in routine primary care

In the West, the use of acupuncture treatments has been investigated and evaluated to establish efficacy. In the past there has been quite a problem with trial evaluations of acupuncture treatments, not least because it has not yet been shown how acupuncture works. Nevertheless, more and more data is demonstrating the efficacy of acupuncture treatments, and acupuncture is being recommended for a range of conditions. For instance, a review by the British Medical Acupuncture Society (BMAS) provides details from systematic reviews and meta-analyses where acupuncture improves symptoms for conditions seen in primary care including chronic back pain, chronic headache (tension and migraine), osteoarthritis of the knee, post-operative nausea and vomiting, and fibromyalgia. In general the review identifies increased economic benefit for healthcare providers when acupuncture treatments are provided.[9]

A large systematic review of 27 trials concluded that there is promising evidence that acupuncture can treat dysmenorrhoea; for menopausal symptoms a multi-centre trial showed a significant reduction in hot flushes.[10, 11] Many other trials have also found beneficial results, whilst others haven't, and systematic reviews, have failed to come to a definitive conclusion. We have to wonder why some trials find a statistically significant positive effect, and some trials don't, even when asking the same question and when using the same point prescription. Of course, even when using the same point prescription, each acupuncture treatment is different; the relationship between a doctor and a patient changes, even if the same doctor sees the same patient. And acupuncture is a procedure, not a pill.

Possible mechanisms of action

Acupuncture can alleviate illness and improve health, and researchers are steadily exploring and discovering possible ways by which stimulation of an acupuncture point can influence symptoms of an illness, the possible mechanisms of action. For acupuncture to increase the likelihood of conception, or to benefit symptoms of menopause there must be a physiological change. In addition to other considerations, an excellent review published at the turn of this century[12] explores potential pathways, which include psychological, neurological and neuroendocrinologlical pathways. These technological developments have begun to establish the molecular environment and how it influences health and behaviour. In fact, as technology has increased, so the potential to learn and study biochemistry and organic chemistry has also expanded as never before, and more and more studies are bringing information to the table elucidating potential pathways.

In their review, Anderson and colleagues (2007) suggest four possible methods by which acupuncture could improve IVF outcomes.[13]

1. Modulating neuroendocrinological factors by influencing the hypothalamic–pituitary–ovarian axis (HPO).
2. Increasing blood flow to the uterus and ovaries: both peripheral and cerebral blood flow have been shown to be modulated by acupuncture.[14, 15, 16, 17, 18]
3. Stress, anxiety and depression have a negative correlation with successful IVF outcomes.[19] Treatment with acupuncture has been shown to significantly alleviate depression, anxiety and stress.[20, 21]
4. Acupuncture modulates cytokines, and a range of cytokines are required to ensure optimal uterine receptivity and implantation.[22]

Anderson's review identifies a range of molecules that are modulated by acupuncture, all of which are related to fertility and IVF outcomes. These include leptin,[23] interleukins 1 (IL-1), 1b (IL-1B) and 6,[24, 25, 26] leukemia inhibitory factor (LIF),[27, 28] and nitric oxide and nitric oxide synthases.[29, 30] In addition, other trials using functional magnetic resonance imaging (fMRI) and immune response evaluated by leukocytes, natural killer cells (NK), cytokines, T-cells and B-cells[31, 32, 33] have shown that acupuncture modulates both the central nervous and peripheral nervous systems, suggesting that afferent neuronal stimulation by acupuncture influences hypothalamic adrenergic anti-inflammatory efferent response to mediate the immune system.

In many ways, the effects of acupuncture rely on nociception (de-qi, the sensation of numbness or contraction when an acupuncture point is stimulated). Zijlstra and colleagues put forward a suggested mechanism involving the interrelation of cytokines beginning with the simultaneous release of calcitonin gene related peptide (CGRP), substance P (SP) and b-endorphin at the point of stimulation.[34]

What happens at stimulation? In terms of nervous innervation, investigations have found that in rats significantly increased nerve density was apparent in acupoints, whereas in dogs acupoints were associated with significantly decreased number and density of subcutaneous nerve structures and increased levels of the neurotransmitter associated with pain, substance P.[35, 36] In addition, more recent research found increased levels of signalling molecules, nitric oxide and nitric oxide synthases, an accumulation of calcium, zinc, iron and copper ions, and ultra-fine micro vessels at acupuncture points.[37, 38, 39] The difference in the neurochemical profile between acupuncture points and non-acupuncture points may be one of the reasons why patients experience different sensations in different acupuncture points on stimulation. Sensation relies on signalling (and not derogating from the finding that belief [placebo] also modulates sensation). Nervous innervation may be different between acupuncture points (that may be species specific), which may relate to a difference in cytokine expression. Cytokine expression may explain the difference in tissue reaction and sensation.[40, 41, 42, 43]

Acupuncture achieves a therapeutic effect by a variety of stimuli, including needling, acupressure and electrical stimulation. Research has shown that acupuncture can modulate a range of cytokines and other biochemicals, some of which appear to be required for uterine receptivity and implantation. Currently in the West there is no technique that offers such a variety in the stimulation of nerves, both peripherally and in the brain.

2

Natural Fertility

Section 1: Cycles, conception and hormonal interactions

In the twenty-first-century Western world, the average age of menarche is 12–13 years old. In comparison to previous times, to the middle of the nineteenth century say, where the age of the first menstrual cycle was mid- to late-teens, this decrease in the age of the menarche appears to represent an increase in reproductivity.[1]

The reason for the fall in the average age of menarche might be more due lifestyle factors, such as nutrition, stress and birth weight, than genetic factors, such as mother's age at menarche.[2, 3] Whereas before it would have taken longer to reach the required ratio due to lifestyle, exercise and nutrition, now increased living standards in the West probably bear some responsibility for a decline in exercise, and increased consumption of fast food and other highly processed consumables rich in sodium, salt and sugar.[4] Early menarche is an established indicator of a higher risk of breast cancer[5] and is linked to metabolic disorders and disease in adulthood. Mortality is also increased. There is evidence that the life span of women whose menarche arrived early is also shorter.[6]

Natural reproduction is a cycle, and all cycles fluctuate, rising and falling. A healthy cycle will fluctuate within a range that ensures its purpose is fulfilled. On average, the given length of a menstrual cycle is 28 days. However, natural cycles between 25 and 35 days are still normal, and it is usual to see a variation of four days in any natural cycle. If the cycle varies significantly more than four days, by eight days or more, it is considered irregular.

Cycles and reproduction also vary according to seasons, although less so in the developed world, due to more privileged lifestyles. There is also a natural decline in the ability to become pregnant. On average we are looking at a woman's age of 35 when fertility begins to decline, although the decline progresses at a geometric rate, not an exponential rate, and has more to do with ovarian age than cycle regularity. Cycles begin to become significantly more irregular at the time of perimenopause and eventually cease altogether after the menopause. Menstrual cycles will continue until menopause, the average age for which is 50.

So the natural ability to become pregnant is cyclical. There is a beginning and an end from menarche to menopause; there are variations each month in the menses; and variations in the ability to become pregnant according to seasons and lifestyle.

The cycle is biphasic. These two phases are quite distinct in character and purpose, and the biochemistry of a woman is significantly different in these two phases. The initial phase – the follicular phase – begins at day one of the menstrual cycle, when the menstrual bleed starts. As the name suggests, the follicular phase is the time when the follicles grow and the uterus begins to prepare itself for an embryo. It ends at the time of ovulation. The second phase – the luteal phase – is also called the secretory stage; here, the uterus becomes receptive to embryo implantation and the follicle that has released the egg, the oocyte, metamorphoses into an entirely new construct.

The processes of the cycle, the inter-variation of the reproductive glands, hormones and neurohormones, and the changes of structure in the reproductive organs are managed by an internal axis. Medicine, both modern and from a TCM point of view, broadly understands fertility in terms of an axis, the fertility axis. In TCM thought the fertility axis relates to the interrelations between organ functions. In modern medicine the fertility axis is the relationship between the hypothalamus, the pituitary and the ovaries, and is studied in the fields of physiology, gynaecology and endocrinology. It is often referred to as the hypothalamus–pituitary–gonadal axis or the hypothalamus–pituitary–ovarian (HPO) axis.

Another important relationship that has a bearing on fertility is the hypothalamus–pituitary–adrenal gland axis (HPA), which reflects the stress we are experiencing and have experienced in our lives, and is discussed in Chapter 6.

The healthy functioning of the hypothalamus is exceptionally important. It has direct and indirect relationships with the reward system relating to feeding and habits, the autonomic and central nervous systems, body temperature and endocrine systems. Including hormones and neurotransmitters related to reproduction, it secretes or causes the secretion of a range of chemicals that are directly related to behaviour and attachment. These include the stress hormones cortisol, adrenalin and noradrenalin, and oxytocin. Sleep and the circadian rhythms are key for a healthy functioning hypothalamus. It is a highly sensitive organ and responds to many stimuli that are directly involved in reproduction.

In reproduction, the hypothalamus works with the pituitary gland. Both the hypothalamus and the pituitary gland are located in the brain. In addition to their other responsibilities, they influence the uterus and ovaries, although of that pair, the ovaries have the greatest role. The ovaries in turn provide feedback to the hypothalamus and so influence the hypothalamus directly in the HPO axis. Since the function of the hypothalamus is directly influenced by the reproductive axis it is quite natural to assume that the reproductive axis also indirectly influences many other systems that the hypothalamus governs.

Fertility relationships

A primary role of the hypothalamus and pituitary gland is to guide reproductivity. They send messages to the ovaries and without the correct administration of this function, reproduction will become inhibited, irregular and will ultimately fail.

In their turn, the ovaries and uterus adapt to the messages, and feed back to the hypothalamus and pituitary gland to let them know what has happened and how they have adapted. The hypothalamus and pituitary gland respond to this feedback by modulating their messages, and signal back to the ovaries, but this time the messages are changed in volume and frequency to accommodate how the ovaries have reacted.

The main signalling method used is endocrinological; the main messages sent are hormones and neurohormones. The main hormones involved are oestrogens and progesterone, gonadotropin-releasing hormone (GnRH), follicle-stimulating hormone (FSH), and luteinising hormone (LH). Oestrogen is actually a collective noun, under which three forms are associated in non-pregnant cycling women: oestrone, oestriol and oestradiol (the fourth form, oestetrol, is only produced during pregnancy). The main oestrogen in naturally cycling non-pregnant women is oestradiol.

The reproductive cycle

The beginning of the reproductive cycle is called the follicular phase. At the beginning of the cycle there is comparatively little oestrogen. Oestrogen is produced mostly by cells within the follicles, called granulosa cells. At the beginning of the menstrual cycle there is a deficit of oestrogen because at the beginning of the cycle the follicles are dormant.

The hypothalamus recognises the oestrogen deficit. As a result of the low levels of oestrogen, it is able to increase the production and secretion of GnRH. The pituitary gland receives the GnRH and is stimulated by it. It produces and secretes FSH, which stimulates follicular growth and also starts maturing oocytes. The pituitary also begins to produce and secrete LH.

The ovaries receive these messages and adapt. The volume of FSH encourages the growth of a clutch of follicles. As the follicles grow, they become receptive to LH. The larger they grow, the more receptive they become. Towards the end of the follicular phase a dominant follicle, the Graafian follicle, will arise (although in some cases in natural fertility, more than one follicle may become dominant, in IVF it's normal to attempt to acquire more than one), and the rest of the clutch will subside and be subsumed into the ovary.

No longer dormant, the follicles also begin to increase production of oestrogen. Oestrogen has an inhibiting effect on the production of GnRH. GnRH is required to stimulate the secretion of FHS and LH. As oestrogen levels increase, so the amount of GnRH decreases which concomitantly decreases secretion of FSH. The amount of oestrogen produced relates to the volume and frequency of the FSH received from the pituitary.

The uterus picks up the oestrogen message and also starts to respond, preparing for an embryo by changing the nature and morphology of the endometrium and thickening the endometrium.

With the emergence of the Graafian follicle things start to change again. The dominant follicle, initially approximately 10mm in diameter starts to grow more rapidly and secretes more oestrogen. It begins to swell with follicular fluid, which is a source of a number of significant constituents important for the developing oocyte, including cytokines, gonadotropins, prolactin and hyaluronan.[7] The receptors that enable the follicle to receive LH also increase in both number and capacity.

The hypothalamus recognises the increase in oestrogen. This feedback inhibits production of GnRH, so the hypothalamus increases the pulse frequency. The rapid increase in oestrogen causes the GnRH pulses to increase dramatically over a very short period of time, which leads to a sudden surge in LH. The sudden surge in LH causes the follicle to rupture and release its charge into the waiting fimbriae (from the Latin, meaning fringe or border) of the fallopian tube.

A slightly more in depth look at the process is as follows: the hypothalamus secretes GnRH to the anterior pituitary, causing the anterior pituitary to produce and secrete both FSH and LH. FSH starts the maturation of the follicles and stimulates the maturation of germ cells, which become gametes. A gamete (originally derived from the Greek *gamos*, meaning marry) is a cell type that is distinct from other cells in that it is a reproductive precursor. Other words for a gamete are oocyte, ovum, egg and sperm. A gamete of one sex will combine with a gamete from the opposite sex to form an embryo.

Ovulation

The follicular cycle continues. The Graafian follicle continues to grow, swelling with follicular fluid and becoming more receptive to LH. At the same time it is producing oestrogen, so the growth spurt results in a large increase in oestrogen, which suppresses the production of GnRH. The hypothalamus responds by switching to another delivery method and increases the frequency of pulses. It is this dramatic increase in frequency that causes the sudden surge in LH. The surge lasts for 24 to 48 hours during which time the dominant follicle ruptures. The rupturing follicle triggers a change in the cycle.

A mature egg is freed to begin its journey. The dominant follicle metamorphoses, changing shape, function and form, and becomes the corpus luteum. It starts to produce progesterone and in so doing initiates the luteal phase.

The luteal phase

The egg has been released into the fallopian tube. The follicle metamorphoses and becomes the corpus luteum. The corpus luteum begins to produce progesterone.

The influence of progesterone

When the dominant follicle ruptures, a whole host of changes occur because a woman's body begins preparing for an embryo.

One of the critical changes is the production of progesterone. Whereas before the follicle provided containment and provision of a nurturing essence for the maturing oocyte, in rupturing the follicle metaphoses into the corpus luteum, a structure to help prepare the environment that a potential embryo will enter.

The corpus luteum begins to produce progesterone. Progesterone is a warming invigorator and many women are able to feel this physically. On temperature readings charted on a basal body temperature chart it should be readily observable.

During the follicular phase, the inner lining of the uterus, the endometrium, has steadily thickened. Under the influence of progesterone it becomes secretory. Glands begin to grow, secreting a wide range of substances that will influence the embryo and support implantation. In addition to this the luminal epithelium grown during the follicular phase also changes. Epithelial tissue is one of the four basic tissue types and is present in many muscosal cavities. Since epithelial cells are 'avascular', that is, without blood vessels, they rely on sustenance from a basement membrane. The term epithelium is derived from the Greek *epi*, meaning 'on' or 'upon', and *thele*, meaning 'nipple'. Luminal means a central cavity in a tube or tubular organ or cell.

The egg

During its time in the follicle, the oocyte has been nourished by the fluid the follicle has been producing to aid its maturation. Once released, the oocyte begins to travel down the fallopian tubes. Here in the fallopian tubes it will meet the sperm that will fertilise it. At the point of conception both egg and sperm cease to exist and become a unique, single cell organism of 46 chromosomes, the technical term for which is a zygote (meaning to 'join' or to 'yoke'). At the end of the first week it is then referred to as an embryo (from the Greek, meaning 'young one') and remains as such until implantation. However, rarely are these technical terms retained now; in general the term 'zygote' is dropped in favour of the term 'embryo'.

Whilst the embryo grows, at the very beginning of life its size does not increase; only the number of cells increases. At around day three or four the embryo has evolved to 12 cells or more. An embryo at this stage is called a 'morula'. The word 'morula' is derived from Latin and means 'mulberry', because the embryo at this stage looks like a mulberry. It continues to divide and on day five post-ovulation undergoes a significant transition. It forms a hollow sphere of cells, called a blastula or blastocyst. Its outer surface becomes the trophectoderm, which will become the external epithelial layer of the placenta, whilst the inner cell mass (ICM) is formed within. The cells in the ICM are pluripotent stem cells. Implantation can only happen when the embryo has reached the blastocyst stage.

Embryo implantation

From the moment of ovulation and the formation of the corpus luteum, progesterone has begun its work to prepare the uterus for implantation. Thickened during the follicular phase, the endometrium becomes secretory, glandular, and the luminal epithelium begins to change. Seven days after ovulation, the endometrium has matured and is ready to receive the embryo. This stage in the cycle evolution is called the 'window of implantation'.

There is a body of evidence suggesting that the preferred site of blastocyst attachment to the endometrium are structures that are only grown during the early stages of progesterone secretion. Originally these were named pinopods. However, due to the differences between animals and humans, they have recently been renamed uterodomes. [8, 9, 10] Uterodomes have been found not only in the window of implantation, but also throughout the luteal cycle and so their role as a marker of endometrial receptivity has yet to be confirmed.[11]

Uterodomes have several known functions. They are pinocytotic, literally drawing in uterine fluid. It is thought that in doing so, the volume of the uterus is reduced, which means that the walls of the uterus are drawn closer to the embryo. The growth of uterodomes is inhibited by oestrogen. There is also a strong correlation between the presence of LIF and uterodomes, and their development appears to be significantly hindered when LIF is not present.[12] It is interesting to note that the absence of LIF also significantly impairs pregnancy.

In natural fertility, the blastocyst enters the womb six or seven days after ovulation. In a text-book 28-day cycle this is around day 20 or 21 and is in the middle of the luteal phase. This is the window of implantation, the point at which the endometrium is prepared to receive the blastocyst, and in general it lasts four days. In this type of cycle, implantation occurs between seven and nine days after ovulation. Where cycles vary, it is important to chart the progress of the cycle using a basal body temperature chart (BBT).

The endometrium has evolved to prepare for implantation, and now the secretions also change in nature. Iron and fat-soluble vitamins are secreted, as well as proteins, cholesterol, steroids and other smaller molecules that are necessary for implantation.

On entering the uterus the blastocyst is already beginning to hatch. The blastocyst and uterus begin a sequence that is called 'cross talk'. Cross talk is the dialogue that occurs between the blastocyst and the endometrium or, to use the scientific expression, the 'maternal interface'. This dialogue only occurs during the window of implantation, and it is chemical in nature.

The process of implantation involves three stages: apposition, adhesion and invasion.

APPOSITION

The blastocyst positions itself close to the endometrial wall and forms a loose attachment, known as tethering. This is the process of apposition. The fluid inside the blastocyst has steadily been increasing, causing its membrane, the zona pellucida, to expand and rupture, allowing the blastocyst to hatch.

Hatching causes the secretion of signalling molecules to flow out, signalling the status of the blastocyst. Research suggests that these messages may also influence its position. To form an attachment, the blastocyst must place its most receptive and communicative part as close as possible to the most receptive/communicative part of the endometrium. The most communicative part of the blastocyst is the rupture from which so many messages are coming. On the maternal side, it is unclear which part of the endometrium is the most communicative, but other literature suggests that as well as uterodomes, the preferred place of attachment might be areas of inflammation.

ADHESION

Adhesion is when the ties between the embryo and the endometrium become much stronger and the blastocyst begins to become physically attached. At the time of adhesion, communication between the blastocyst and the endometrium is significantly increased. The cells that surround the blastocyst, are called 'trophoblasts'. These specialised cells begin to slough off the blastocyst and to burrow into the endometrium, seeking secure footings. These cells form the external epithelial layer of the placenta.

INVASION

The trophoblasts grow in number. With this increase, the tentative foothold established at the end of the appostion state and at the beginning of the time of adhesion is enlarged, not only in the surrounding area but deeper into the endometrium as the trophoblasts extend their hold. It is during this time that we can say true implantation is initiated and placentation has begun.

Placentation

The word 'placenta' has several origins. I prefer 'little mother' or 'grandmother' from pre-Roman literature rather than the more prosaic Greek descriptive, 'slab-like'.

The burrowing trophoblasts are intent on reaching the base layer of the uterus. As they pursue this goal, they change and merge. The boundaries between the cells 'dissolve' and they become a single cell mass that surrounds the burgeoning placenta. The process of burrowing continues as the trophoblasts actively invade the uterine wall until the embryo is firmly embedded in the endometrium. The invasion establishes the pathways that provide nutrients to the embryo from the mother. The placenta continues to grow throughout pregnancy. However, the first 12 to 13 weeks see the most rapid growth and the pregnancy is still at risk during this time.

Section 2: Molecular interactions

One of the keys to embryo implantation is embryo–mother cross talk. Cross talk relies on both the mother and the embryo being able to recognise a signal and receive it, and to pass the signal on. In terms of embryo implantation and cell signalling pathways whereby extracellular molecules transfer information to the interior of a cell, this process is the domain of molecular interactions, neuroendocrinology and molecular medicine.

Molecular medicine seeks to understand disease and pathogenesis at the molecular level. It differs from genetic medicine insofar as the latter researches disease origins at the hereditary level and seeks to treat them using genetic technology.

As a discipline, molecular medicine is not quite 65 years old and essentially is birthed from studies in haemoglobin. The first paper that truly established a molecular basis of disease was published in 1949. Written by one the greatest scientists of the twentieth century, Linus Pauling, and his colleagues, the paper demonstrated that sickle cell anaemia is based on a genetic condition.[13] This paper also established Pauling's concept that molecular disease causes evolutionary adaptation.

The Emeritus Professor Roger Williams, who discovered the vitamin pantothenic acid in 1933 and developed a nutritional approach as a treatment of alcoholism, was a contemporary of

Pauling's. Published in 1956, his book *Biochemical Individuality*[14] harks back to Archibald Garrod's work *The Inborn Factors in Disease*, which was published in 1931.[15] Both Garrod and Williams argued for the individuality of human biochemistry and promulgated molecular treatments as a therapeutic approach. Interestingly, both Pauling and Williams focused on natural and nutritional substances for preventative medicine, and in the treatment of molecular conditions.

Molecular medicine progressed at a very slow pace and it was not until the 1970s with the development of the ability to isolate messenger RNA (mRNA) that advancement in this field truly began to evolve. Nevertheless, the lack of technology hampered investigation. For instance, endothelin, the potent vasoconstrictor that is involved in both the HPA and the HPO, and is implicated in follicular growth, was not discovered until the end of the 1980s.[16, 17]

The term 'signalling pathway' is an abbreviation of the term 'signal transduction pathway'. Transduction is derived from the Latin *trans*, meaning 'across' or 'go beyond', and *ducere*, 'to lead'. The combination forms *traducere,* meaning 'change over', 'lead across' or 'convert'.

Signal transduction arises from the work of the Nobel Prize winner Martin Rodbell, whose theory that biological signalling could be analogous to the technological signalling being developed in computer science drove him to elucidate the process of transduction in the late 1960s and early 1970s. The term itself is derived from an article Rodbell wrote in 1980.[18]

Signal transduction cascade

Humans process and communicate information, internally and externally. At the internal level, a cell needs to process, and is capable of processing, information from outside the cell body to within it in order to adapt. For instance, a cell may receive information of temperature changes from extracellular signalling molecules. If heat suddenly becomes excessive, the cell will synthesise proteins to protect itself from harm.

Receptors are molecules that receive extracellular signals. Many cellular receptors are transmembrane: they are bound within the membrane of the cell. They have an exterior presentation on the surface of the cell, and an interior presentation within the cell body. When a signalling molecule binds to a transmembrane receptor, the receptor is activated. The activation causes the aspect of the receptor within the cell body to change, to convert, adapt or traduce the signal. The adapted form transmits a signal that triggers a cascade of events; an enzyme is activated, which causes the subsequent activation and change in a second tier of enzymes, and so on, until the cascade achieves the activation of the appropriate enzymes that forms the response of the cell. An example of a transmembrane protein is the glycoprotein 130 (gp130).

Glycoproteins

Glycoproteins are involved in cell-to-cell signalling, and are often transmembrane proteins. They are deeply involved in the immune system and interact with a type of white blood cell called a lymphocyte. The word 'lymphocyte' originates from the Greek 'goddess of clear spring water *Nymphe*', and was modified in Latin to *lympha* to mean 'clear water, or a goddess of water'. It was employed in 1725 to denote the clear fluid found in the body.

Glycoproteins are important for the immune system and white blood cells. They also interact specifically with T-cells through a cellular mediator called the major histocompatibility complex (MHC). They can be found in the zona pellucida and are important for fertilisation, in collagen for binding tissue and different tissue types, and for taste recognition. Other examples of glycoproteins include the hormones FSH and human chorionic gonadotropin (hCG).

Lymphocytes

Three main types of lymphocytes exist: large molecules called natural killer cells (NK), which are the focus of intense investigation in fertility, and the smaller two molecules, t and b lymphocytes. Both T and B lymphocytes are cells of the system of aqcuired immunity, the adaptive immune response. This is the immune response that learns and remembers the shape and form of pathogens. Whereas the B-cells make antibodies to bind antigens, T-cells do not make antibodies but among their other functions generate cytotoxic cells to destroy infected cells.

T-cells acquired the name because they are matured in the immune system organ, the thymus. The thymus is situated directly behind the sternum at the level of the Conception Channel point, Shan Zhong, Ren 17. Although B-cells are generated in the bone marrow of mammals, the denotation is actually derived from their origin of discovery, the bursa of Fabricius, a specialised organ for the development of B-cells in birds.

Cytokines

Glycoprotein 130 is a critical component of the transmembrane receptors that are known as type 1 cytokine receptors. It is the recent tremendous interest cytokines have generated that has necessitated the classification of cytokine receptors into groups based on their shape and structure.

The signals that receptors receive are chemical. Hormones are signalling molecules, as are neurotransmitters. The immune system also uses signalling molecules, called cytokines. The word 'cytokine' is derived from the Greek words *cyto*, meaning cell, and *kinos*, meaning movement. A cytokine is released by a cell to influence the activity of another cell. It's worth noting at this point that some cytokines are referred to as hormones, and some are also known as neurotransmitters. Some cytokines are important during the luteal phase, some are important during the window of implantation, and in terms of reproduction, leptin, also known as the anti-obesity molecule, is important throughout the entire cycle.

Some cytokines are absolutely critical for embryo implantation, placentation and a healthy pregnancy; if they are not present at all, or not within a healthy range, implantation will fail, or the pregnancy will fail, or foetal growth will be endangered. Most of these exceptionally small chemicals are multi-purpose and interact with other systems in our wonderfully complex body.

All type 1 cytokine receptors are transmembrane, that is, they are bound within the membrane of a cell, providing an exterior and interior presentation on the membrane. Type 1 cytokine receptors co-relate with cytokines that are understood to be involved in the regulation of the immune system and the cellular blood component systems, called haematopoietic systems. Hence the reason that type 1 cytokine receptors are also known as haematopoietin receptors.[19]

Examples of this super family of receptors are interleukins; LIF, which is also a member of the interleukin 6 family; erythopoietin, which is involved in the production of blood; and prolactin, which contributes to the regulation of the immune system, the sexual refractory period, lactation, blood, angiogenesis and in the production of myelin.

Signalling pathways: STAT3, JAK STAT, endocrine, paracrine and autocrine

Signalling pathways are required to transmit information. In addition to STAT3 and JAK STAT, many other signalling pathways have been identified, including the MAPK (mitogen-activated protein kinases) pathways, which are implicated in both trophoblastic invasion and cervical ripening, and the Hedgehog pathway, which is important for embryogenesis.

STAT 3

The signal transducer and activator of transcription 3, or STAT3, is a protein that controls the transcription of genetic data from DNA to mRNA. Transcription is the process whereby DNA makes RNA through mRNA. STAT3, then, is a transcription factor.

STAT3 is known to relate to certain interleukins such as LIF, which activates it, interferons and leptin. It is also thought that STAT3 is critically involved in embryo implantation,[20] pregnancy and auto immune diseases.[21, 22, 23]

A healthy STAT3 signalling pathway is required for fertility. When STAT3 is impaired, obesity can occur, which is a major cause of infertility and other significant diseases, and the LH surge can be blocked. When it is not present at all, both obesity and infertility occur.[24]

JAK (JANUS KINASE) STAT

The JAK STAT signalling pathway consists of a receptor, a Janus Kinase and a STAT. The name Janus is the name of the two-faced Roman god and is used to denote its unique structure.

In order to transduce the signal they receive, molecules such as prolactin or cytokines, including the haematopoietin family, need to be able to instruct an on–off switch in intercellular proteins.

Yet they have no catalytic ability because they lack a compound that can phosphorylate energy to a specific substance within a cell. This means a biocatalyst is required to transfer a phosphate group from a molecule that contains an abundance of phosphate, such as adenosine triphosphate (ATP), to another molecule. The type of substance that can do this is a particular enzyme, called a kinase, and in the case of the JAK STAT pathway the enzyme tyrosine kinase. Tyrosine (tyrosine is derived from the Greek, meaning 'cheese') is a non-essential amino acid that cells use to synthesise proteins. A tyrosine kinase is an enzyme that functions as an on–off switch by transferring phosphate to a specific protein in a cell. The phosphorylation of the protein is the chemical on–off switch. Inhibition of the JAK STAT signalling pathway is now the focus of clinical attention to treat psoriasis, rheumatoid arthritis and other conditions.[25, 26]

THE ENDOCRINE PATHWAYS

Within endocrinology there are five main pathways: endocrine, intracrine, juxtacrine, paracrine and autocrine.

'Endocrine' is derived from the Greek words *endon*, meaning 'internal', and *krinein*, meaning 'from', 'secrete' or 'separate'. Endocrine signalling is the province of endocrinologists.

Endocrine glands employ signalling molecules such as hormones. Hormones act on cells that are some distance from their origin. An example of this is the glycoprotein FSH which originates in the anterior pituitary and stimulates follicular growth on the ovary.

In contradistinction, the paracrine pathway relates to signalling that occurs between neighbouring cells, conferred by cytokines, or local hormones, which are also known as paracrine hormones. Paracrine is from the Greek *para*, meaning 'near' or 'side by side', and *krinein* as mentioned above. Paracrine signalling is similar to endocrine signalling, but since paracrine ligands do not enter the blood, paracrine signalling usually occurs between cells of the same tissue type that work so closely together they are almost one unit. Nerve impulses are a good example of this signalling pathway. The transmission of a nerve impulse, the action potential, causes the nerve cell to secrete a neurotransmitter. The neurotransmitter crosses the synaptic gap and binds with its receptor on the neighbouring nerve cell, transmitting the message, the action potential, to its neighbour.

'Auto' comes from the Greek *autos*, meaning 'self' or 'same' or 'one's self'. Autocrine therefore refers to self-cellular reactions. This means that cells respond to the reactions and substances they produce themselves. A specific signalling molecule will be received on the appropriate receptor. The receptor will become activated and the activation confluents through the receptor and changes the aspect of it that is presented on the inner surface of the cell membrane. This will then transmit the specific message to the inner cell mass, which causes a signal transduction cascade.

Neuromodulators of fertility and implantation

The field of neuroendocrinology is relatively new, and sophisticated technologies to investigate these substances have only recently been engineered. The recent rapid increase in sophistication and range of technologies means that it is much easier to explore these chemicals and their interactions, and the pace in their development means that new molecules and novel interactions are being discovered all the time.

Implantation relies on a range of factors. Results of investigations seem to suggest that the molecules present during the window of implantation are more pro-inflammatory than neutral or anti-inflammatory. There has also been a theory that some cytokines are key to implantation, for example LIF and interleukin 11 (IL-11).

The blastocyst must orient itself to the endometrium. This process of orientation, called apposition, is based on polarity. At this time, the way that polarity is established and how the blastcyst is able to be oriented is thought to involve the inflammatory response, cytokines and chemokines.

There is some evidence that blastocysts prefer scar tissue as sites of implantation.[27] Scar tissue in the uterus originates from Caesarean section in the main, although other endometrial surgery may also cause scarring. There is also a relatively new treatment in IVF called pipelle where a small local injury in the endometrium is purposefully created, which, its proponents suggest, may improve implantation.[28]

Scar tissue is a focal point of inflammation. As such it will be secreting inflammatory cells and signalling molecules, such as cytokines and an even more specialised group of cytokines, chemokines. In the uterine milieu, chemokines play several roles, which include the regulation of T helper cells, Th1 and Th2, at sites of potential infection. Some evidence suggests that it is these signalling molecules that manage the apposition of the blastocyst to the endometrium. However, the embryo is essentially a foreign body and one of the functions of the immune system is to reject foreign bodies, yet in many cases implantation succeeds. Recently it has been shown that at the time of implantation, immune recruiting chemokines in the decidua are silenced, thereby preventing T-cell cytotoxic activity.[29]

Also involved in apposition are adhesion molecules, such as the glycoproteins, selectins. Selectins are cell surface molecules, and belong to a system of identification and classification of cell surface molecules. The identification protocol is the CD nomenclature, the 'cluster of differentiation' or 'cluster of designation' (CD). In humans, more than 350 clusters of differentiation have been identified so far (the full list of clusters of differentiation is available online[30]). Selectins (E, L and P selectins) are numbered cluster of differentiation 62 (CD62). They are involved in many of the cellular responses to homeostasis and adaptation, and are significantly involved in acute and chronic inflammatory processes.[31] Inflammation causes cytokines and tumour necrosis factor alpha (TNFα) to stimulate the secretion of selectins from cells, a process employed in blastocyst apposition and adhesion.[32, 33]

Cytokines involved in implantation

One of the pathways by which acupuncture works may be through the inflammatory response. Cytokines involved in the inflammatory response and that have been modulated by acupuncture include the IL-1 and IL-6 super families, leukemia inhibitory factor (LIF) and leptin.

INTERLEUKIN 1 (IL-1)

Interleukin 1 (IL-1) is a pro-inflammatory cytokine. Its effects on inflammation can be inhibited by its antagonist, interleukin 1 receptor antagonist (IL-1Ra), which is produced by another pro-inflammatory molecule involved in implantation, tumour necrosis factor alpha (TNFα). However, IL-Ra is likely to cause arrested development when peri-implantation blastocysts secrete it.

IL-1 is present throughout the menstrual cycle, and because of this it is conjectured that IL-1 may also influence other stages of pre-pregnancy and implantation events, such as fallopian tube activity during the embryo transition from the fimbriae to uterus. During the window of implantation, IL-1 stimulates the endometrial production and secretion of leukemia inhibitory factor, and the production of leptin and its receptor OB-R.[34, 35]

IL-1 receptor 1 (IL-1R1), IL-1b and IL-1 receptor a (IL-1Ra) are expressed by blastocysts. In response to IL-1 stimulation, blastocysts secrete hCG and IL-1.[36, 37] During implantation, blastocyst IL-1 binds with receptors on the endometrium. Blastocyst IL-1 acts in concert with maternally secreted IL-1 to increase expression of the adhesion molecule integrin beta, which plays an important role in adhesion, and to a lesser extent during apposition.

INTERLEUKIN 6 (IL-6)

The IL-6 family of cytokines plays a highly important role in implantation. All members of this family signal through the glycoprotein gp130 and some activate the STAT3 signalling pathway.[38] These include LIF, interleukin 6 (IL-6) and interleukin 11 (IL-11). Both LIF and IL-6 are pro-inflammatory cytokines, whereas IL-11 is anti-inflammatory.

IL-6 is mostly produced by the endometrial epithelium and stromal cells at the time of implantation. Levels of IL-6 are relatively low in the follicular phase and are highest during the window of implantation. IL-6 is controlled by IL-1 and gonadotropin steroid hormones, particularly oestrogen which induces IL-6 expression. Receptors for IL-6 can be found on the endometrium, on the trophoblasts and on the blastocyst. The blastocyst regulates the uterine environment by secreting hCG, which increases secretion of LIF and decreases secretion of IL-6. This means that the inflammatory state of the uterine environment is controlled by both the mother and the blastocyst.

In patients suffering from recurrent miscarriage, serum levels drawn from the peripheral blood were found to have higher than normal levels of IL-6. However, lower than normal IL-6 mRNA has also been found in this group, indicating that a particular range of IL-6 is required.[39]

Leukemia inhibitory factor (LIF)

A member of the interleukin 6 group of cytokines, the pro-inflammatory cytokine LIF is a glycoprotein known to be critical for implantation.[40, 41]

LIF signalling is triggered by the binding of its receptor to gp130. Signal transduction relies on the activation of several signalling pathways including JAK STAT and STAT3.[42, 43] The current progression in the investigations of LIF suggest that it is a molecular mediator between the endometrium, immune cells and trophoblasts. Functionally, LIF inhibits cellular differentiation, and it is this function applied to leukemic cells from which its name is derived.

LIF is upregulated by progesterone. The absence of LIF appears to correlate significantly with infertility.[44] Although it has been found that a low level of LIF in the secretory phase appears to improve the chances of successful pregnancy, perhaps reflecting an appropriate inflammatory status of the uterine environment, other studies have found a marked increase in LIF secretion in the mid to late luteal phase.[45, 46] Moreover, the high levels found in the fallopian tube suggest a dual role for LIF: not only implantation, but also embryo development.[47] Furthermore, Aghajanova (2003) found the presence of LIF to correlate with uterodomes expression whilst it has also been found that where LIF is absent, uterodomes also fail to develop and it is suggested that this may be one of reasons that the absence of LIF causes implantation failure.[48, 49]

LEPTIN

Originally leptin was known as the anti-obesity molecule because of its ability to manage energy and energy stores. However, it is now better understood as an energy reporter and a cytokine, and it is sometimes identified as a hormone.[50] It is secreted by white fat cells, which are known as adipocytes and which are found around the waist and in breast tissue. The larger the number of adipocytes, the more leptin is secreted. In many cases, the hypothalamus detects the rise in leptin and signals to reduce the desire to feed but to increase the desire to exercise. Similarly, when there are insufficient energy stores the hypothalamus detects the decrease in leptin and signals the need to feed and rest.

Leptin appears to be critical for implantation.[51] Appropriate energy stores are critical for fertility. In women, less than 10 per cent of body fat causes a cessation of ovulation and in many cases hypothalamic hypogonadism[52, 53] On the other hand, being overweight and obesity cause infertility and it may be that one of the causes in people suffering from obesity is that obesity simulates a state of negative energy balance.[54, 55]

Oestrogen also appears to regulate weight, food intake and exercise.[56, 57] A deficiency in oestrogen causes leptin insensitivity, and in chronic oestrogen deficiency, leptin resistance.[58] Since elevated levels of leptin inform the hypothalamus that there is a surfeit of stored energy, the hypothalamus should cease signalling the requirement to feed and the person with leptin insensitivity or leptin resistance would naturally get slimmer. The obverse is true, however. Elevated leptin levels can in fact lead to weight gain, obesity and infertility.

Leptin and its receptor, OB-R, are expressed in the human endometrium and on the embryo. Intracellular signalling occurs through the JAK STAT and the MAKP signalling pathways. Animals which are leptin deficient are also infertile. Fertility can be restored, however, by the administration of exogenous leptin.[59]

3

Understanding IVF Part 1

The world population is now just over seven billion and is projected to be just over nine billion within 40 years.[1] By 2007 the worldwide demand for assistance with reproduction was growing at around 9 per cent a year.[2] In 2008, the European Society for Human Reproduction and Embryology (ESHRE) reported a 7.9 per cent increase in demand, and in the UK the Human Fertilisation and Embryology Authority (HFEA) reports a year on year increase in demand for assisted reproduction, with a 4.3 per cent increase from 2010 to 2011.[3,4]

Assisted reproduction technology (ART) is a sub-discipline of gynaecology. ART is emerging as the dominant field in gynaecology and its range and capacity to assist couples are expanding at a pace that is extraordinary. Whilst ART has been growing and expanding, gynaecology as a discipline has been shrinking; there are now surgical procedures from 30 years ago that are obsolete. Some skills, interventions and surgical procedures are being made obsolete as new training and technologies emerge. It is also true to say that specialist medical staff diminish in numbers as a result of this decline.

The agency that regulates and oversees ART in the UK is the Human Fertilisation and Embryology Authority (HFEA). The Canadian equivalent is Assisted Human Reproduction Canada (AHRC). In America clinics can choose to become a member of a governing body, such as the American Society for Reproductive Medicine (ASRM), or the Society for Assisted Reproductive Technologies (SART), but a state-sponsored regulator is absent.

ART covers a range of techniques and treatments to help patients suffering from sub-fertility, and in vitro fertilisation (IVF) is only one, albeit the one that receives most attention. When speaking of patients we should remember that a couple is a patient as much as a single person.

Assisted reproduction

It's usual to take steps when pregnancy is not occurring naturally. It's a process of scaling up interventions. Initially, lifestyle changes will be made, then choosing different options that are passed on through the family's oral tradition, or found on the internet or in the press. A patient may also start seeking, or better yet, already have sought advice from a professional, a specialist not directly related to fertility, a personal trainer perhaps or a nutritional therapist or a yogi or yogini who will provide expert guidance from their field. If those options are insufficient, clinical intervention and the use of assisted reproduction technologies will begin to be explored.

If there is already a clear reason why a patient cannot get pregnant, such as a salpingectomy, where the fallopian tubes have been removed, or an ineffective vasectomy reversal, then these initial steps will still be useful but may also be avoided and the patient will move directly to IVF. There are other reasons why the use of ART may be indicated, for instance, to try to exclude a gene to avoid a hereditary disease, or to inhibit the transfer of a disease such as AIDS.

Allopathic medicine

The term allopathic is derived from the Greek *allos*, meaning 'other' and *patheia*, which means 'suffering' and can also mean 'feeling'. Allopathic refers to a system of medicine that treats a symptom or disease using a remedy that causes an opposite effect to the disease or symptom. Essentially, fighting fire with water. Both Western medicine and traditional Chinese herbal medicine are allopathic.

Improving fertility by using fertility medications, also known as fertility drugs, is limited by the number available. Currently very few exist. Gonadotropins, either recombinant (artificial) or derived from a natural source to stimulate the ovary, or hCG are often used to induce ovulation. Stimulating follicular growth by inhibiting oestrogen to increase the secretion of FSH is also often used. The type of pharmaceutical used in this type of treatment is known as a selective oestrogen receptor modulator (SERM). The most well-known preparation in this class is clomiphene.

If these fail, then further intervention will be indicated. Further interventions include intrauterine insemination (IUI) and IVF. By far the most commonly referenced intervention is IVF.

Clomiphene citrate

Clomiphene citrate is marketed under the names Clomid, Omifin and Androxal. It increases production of FSH by inhibiting negative feedback at the hypothalamic level by binding to oestrogen receptors in the hypothalamus. It is used mostly to treat female infertility but sometimes male fertility.

The use of clomiphene is indicated where there is a condition that is preventing ovulation, that is, causing anovulation. In the majority of cases, anovulation is caused by hormonal imbalances. This could be occurring at the hypothalamic level (an estimated 10% of all cases), at the pituitary level, due to a compromised thyroid, or to the impairment of another organ dependent on the hypothalamic–pituitary relationship. It could be due to elevated prolactin secretion, also known as hyperprolactinaemia, which is a normal side effect of breastfeeding and often an unwanted side effect of major tranquillisers inhibiting dopamine secretion. Stress is also known to cause hyperprolactineamia, as are diseases such as Cushing's Disease and acromegaly, and some cancers.

Hormonal dysfunction is at the base of the progression of PCOS, which is also known as Stein Leventhal Syndrome, and there is evidence that it is hereditary.[5] PCOS is probably the most common endocrine disorder and accounts for 90 per cent of anovulatory cases.

Strictly speaking, a follicle is a cyst, and is also called a functional cyst. The word 'cyst' is derived from the Greek *kystis*, meaning a pouch or a bladder. If the follicle does not rupture it can continue to grow. This is called a follicular cyst. On the other hand, if the follicle ruptures it evolves, changes structure and becomes the corpus luteum. In some cases, the rupture closes, and the fluid is retained within the corpus luteum. This is also called a functional cyst. An ovarian cyst is a fluid-filled enclosure on the ovary and in most cases will be benign.

When follicles do not rupture often, the pattern is identified as a syndrome and is called luteinising unruptured follicle syndrome (LUFS). Eventually a large number of unruptured follicles occur on the ovary, and the ovary becomes polycystic. This may then develop into polycystic ovarian syndrome. Polycystic ovarian syndrome is associated with being overweight, hirsutism and infertility.

Administration of clomiphine is known to increase the chances of ovarian cysts.

Gonadotropin treatment for infertility

Gonadotropins are hormones, also known as steroid hormones. The gonadotropins used in fertility treatment to induce ovulation are FSH and LH. These are usually recombinant preparations, that is, artificial. If these fail then a selective oestrogen receptor modulator like clomiphene will be used.

FSH stimulates follicular development. Women have different reactions to this hormone and so most clinics will initially prescribe small doses, which will begin on day three, four or five of the menstrual bleed. Usually, just prior to the beginning of the treatment, the clinic will advise a pelvic ultrasound scan and bloods to check the ovaries for any large cysts and to check hormone levels and then give the go-ahead. The application of gonadotropins is injection under the skin, often into the fat layer in the stomach, in the early evening. Five days after initiation of this treatment, another pelvic ultrasound will be required to check on the number of follicles growing, and bloods will be taken again. The results of these investigations will determine whether there is any change in the amount of FSH that needs to be taken.

The purpose of this treatment is to cause the growth of one or two follicles, between 15 and 18 millimetres at the time of ovulation. If there are three or more then the treatment may be cancelled. To gauge this, regular ultrasounds will be required.

When a follicle has reached a size that indicates a mature egg, hCG will be administered to initiate final maturation of egg and ovulation.

Side effects are possible, as with any treatment. The ovaries are being stimulated and become enlarged, the follicles may be heavy with fluid and so some abdominal discomfort is often reported. Nausea, and in some cases vomiting, may also result. In some cases, gonadotropin treatment for infertility may be converted to a full IVF cycle because the clinician may feel that more control of the cycle is required.

Risks

The main risks are multiple births of either twins or triplets. This type of risk is known to put both mother and babies at risk, and so most clinics take extra care to ensure that the number of follicles is within prescribed limits and the likelihood of this outcome is restricted.

The other main risk is ovarian hyperstimulation syndrome (OHSS). OHSS can occur during IVF treatment with gonadotropins and particularly hCG, and is also seen in early pregnancy but rarely after.

OHSS is mostly mild but it is a complication that is taken seriously because it can become severe and even life threatening. Symptoms include abdominal pain, diarrhoea and a feeling of fullness. Excessive weight gain and thirst, darker urine and vomiting are symptoms of moderate OHSS. Severe symptoms are calf and chest pains, fullness and bloating above the waist and short breath with fluid in the pleura, dark scanty urine, or no urination at all.

Although administration of FSH can lead to OHSS, the prevailing evidence suggests that hCG is the most frequent precipitator, and this is certainly the case in pregnancy where it is the action of hCG on the corpus luteum that causes OHSS.

In IVF treatments, the risk associated with hCG can be alleviated if a GnRH agonist such as buserelin or leuprolide is used, as in the treatment modelled after the 'flare effect'. Essentially, the drug is an artificial preparation that binds to GnRH receptors in the pituitary. Use of this drug can mimic the pre-ovulation events leading to a sudden increase of production and secretion of FSH and LH from the pituitary, called the 'flare effect'.

Intrauterine insemination

Intrauterine insemination (IUI) is an artificial insemination technique. This technology is used when a woman is suffering from sub-fertility and is known to have fully functioning fallopian tubes and a fully functioning uterus. Pathophysiological investigations may have identified male or female factor. In terms of male factor, the deterioration has been significant in the last 50 years, and in the very recent past the decline in male fertility is so dramatic it represents a serious issue.[6,7] For instance, azoospermia, where there are no sperm or where the sperm count is very low, now represents 20 per cent of all male factor sub-fertility[8] and male factor represents 40–50 per cent of all fertility problems.

In female factor, pathophysiology that may indicate the use of IUI includes cervical issues from scarring due to endometriosis or cancer treatments, cervical mucosal issues relating to viscosity or pH balance, or that the woman's immune system has been alerted to the sperm as a foreign and hostile organism. Other areas where IUI is indicated are where there is a communicable disease that would prohibit natural conception, or same-sex relationships.

A cycle of IUI may be stimulated or unstimulated. In addition to OHSS, a stimulated cycle has a higher risk of multiple pregnancies associated with it. Multiple pregnancies carry many dangers for both mother and child (see below). Insofar as this is the case, a couple who require a stimulated cycle will usually be offered IVF instead.

An unstimulated cycle will be monitored, usually with an ovulation kit and often with ultrasound. Once the monitoring begins, the follicle is tracked and as determined by the clinician, hCG will be administered to mature the follicle. When the surge occurs, a catheter is inserted through the cervix and into the womb. Using the catheter, the sperm, previously prepared in the lab, will be transferred into the womb and deposited close to the fallopian tubes, so that the sperm can either meet the egg there or travel to the ampulla (from the Latin, meaning a 'flask' or 'bottle') where fertilisation usually occurs. The actual process of IUI is brief, lasting a few minutes or slightly more, and it takes place at around the same time as the process of natural fertility. This timing depends on the patient's cycle. If the cycle is natural and regular, then the IUI will take place between cycle days 12 and 16.

The National Institute for Clinical Excellence (NICE) Guidelines for 2013 state that IUI should now not be made available on the Health Service in the UK for women who have mild endometriosis, or have been diagnosed with unexplained infertility.[9]

Figures from 2008 published by the HFEA in the UK show that women of 35 years and under who are using this technique can expect almost a 16 per cent chance of being successful.[10] Within five years though, the chances of success drop by more than 60 per cent; statistically, women who are between the ages of 40 and 42 have less than a 5 per cent chance of getting pregnant using this technique.

About IVF

The main treatment for patients who are sub-fertile in ART is in vitro fertilisation (IVF). 'In vitro' is derived from the Latin, meaning 'in a glass', and pertains to the original research that formed the basis of this treatment where fertilisation of the egg occurred in glass Petri dishes.

Origin of IVF

In the US, IVF treatment as a method of reproduction began during the 1930s, in rabbits. Attempts in humans were made in the 1940s and 1960s. In real terms, the history of IVF as a treatment for sub-fertility in humans was established in the UK in 1978 with the birth of the first baby born from this technique, Louise Brown. Her mother Leslie had blocked fallopian tubes and she had been trying to conceive for the preceding nine years. In 1977 consultants took an egg from one of her ovaries and fertilised it with sperm in vitro and transferred the embryo to Lesley's womb.

Following this historic event, consultants in other countries replicated the procedure – in Australia (1980), in the USA (1981) and in Sweden (1982).[11] Since those nascent days the use of IVF has increased significantly.

In general, the numbers of couples requiring IVF in the UK seem to be increasing. Data from the HFEA showing the long-term trends identify a rapid increase between 1992 and 1995. From 1996 until 2006, the numbers of women treated with IVF remained relatively constant, at 18,500.[12] However, in 2006, 34,855 women were treated with 44,275 cycles, resulting in 23.1 per cent live births. In 2007, 36,861 women received 46,829 cycles, resulting in 23.7 per cent live births. In 2007, 39,879 women received 50,687 cycles, an increase of 8.2 per cent. In this last cohort, 24.1 per cent of cycles resulted in a live birth.[13]

The latest data from the HFEA website show that in 2011, 48,147 women had 61,726 cycles of IVF or intracytoplasmic sperm injection (ICSI), from which 17,041 babies were born.[14]

Data between 1978 and 2012 show that, rather than fertility treatment having reached a plateau, it has consistently risen, reflecting an increased need for this discipline. In the 25 years from 1978 to 2003, an estimated two million couples received IVF treatment.[15] From 1991 to 2010 the live birth rate has almost doubled, from 14 per cent to 25 per cent.[16] In eight years, the number of people requiring IVF has doubled: from 2004 to 2012 a further three million people sought IVF.[17] The population in India is 1.22 billion and the latest figures show a rising infertility trend that currently affects about 30 million couples.[18] In spite of the fortunate fact that success rates are increasing, and even though the increase in success rates isn't accelerating as fast as demand, a question that does arise is when, and under what circumstances, will demand for fertility treatment plateau?

Technologies

There are many technologies which are brought to bear in IVF. These include intracytoplasmic sperm injection, assisted hatching, embryo splitting, zygote intrafallopian transfer, cytoplasmic transfer, autologous endometrial coculture, preimplantation genetic diagnosis and sex determination.

The evolution of biological science is extraordinary. Things that were the province of science fiction are now science fact – for example, that it is now possible to offer a treatment that might be able to exclude a gene that causes a hereditary disease, like sickle-cell anaemia.

The types of IVF cycle vary, but the three most common cycles are the long protocol, the short protocol and the natural cycle. In essence, each cycle seeks to replicate the hormonal balance of your natural cycle, but in both the short and long cycles, the levels of hormones used generally exceed those that naturally occur in your body. The main difference between the long and short cycle is that the long cycle closes down a woman's natural cycle. After this has happened both long and short cycles hyperstimulate the ovaries.

What are the costs of IVF?

In the UK, the average cost of IVF is about £5000 to £6000 per cycle, although these figures are really a broad brush.[19] The HFEA point out that in the main, prices are not regulated, but since clinics compete for patients they remain relatively similar.[20] However, prices do differ between clinics and also depend on condition and choice of treatment. Moreover, since the overall national success rate hovers just below 30 per cent the chances weigh against the patient, and so it's likely that more than one cycle will be required. There is a ray of sunshine however. Very recently a new, low-cost treatment option has been developed that could reduce some IVF treatments to just 15 per cent of the current cost.[21, 22]

In the USA, the cost for IVF is around $12,000, depending on clinic and condition. IVF with egg donation is the most costly, with one cycle costing between $25,000 and $30,000.

IVF cycles

The treatments that are brought to bear in IVF range from mundane – if the miracle that IVF is could ever be called mundane! – to extraordinarily ambitious. The cornerstone of IVF is the process upon which each treatment is based, and the cornerstone was laid in 1978. Since then two main cycles have been developed, the long and the short cycle, both of which use gonadotropins to hyperstimulate the ovaries to grow follicles. A third cycle of IVF has recently evolved, called a natural cycle or mild cycle, where very small amounts of gonadotropins are used to gently stimulate the ovaries and grow one or two follicles. The cycles are monitored using ultrasound and blood tests and they all involve catheterisation for embryo transfer. The primary differences in these cycles are the levels of gonadotropins and other drugs used, and diagnosis of genetic pathology that might require a specific treatment approach. For example, pre-genetic diagnosis will require at least three embryos (see Chapter 5). This effectively rules out the natural cycle (not to be confused with a patient's natural cycle) and mild cycles, and clinical advice may also suggest that the long cycle is the most appropriate.

In addition to this, a frozen embryo cycle or a donor egg cycle are slightly different simply because the patient will not be expected to have her ovaries hyperstimulated.

THE LONG CYCLE

The long cycle suppresses the normal menstrual cycle by preventing the pituitary from secreting FSH and LH.

In Chapter 2 we discussed the normal cycle in terms of the relationships between the hypothalamus, the pituitary and the ovaries, the HPO axis. GnRH is released from the hypothalamus to tell the pituitary to release FSH and LH. However, in an IVF cycle, it is often considered optimal to mature quite a few eggs, rather than one or two. Also, the larger the follicle grows, the more receptive it becomes to LH so, if left unregulated, there is a chance that the surge in LH arrives before the clinic is ready.

A GnRH antagonist (such as cetrotide or orgalutron) or agonist (such as buserelin or synarel) may be used. Antagonists are receptor blockers; they bind to receptors and in so doing prevent the target molecule, in this case natural GnRH, from binding to it. The prevention of natural GnRH blocks secretion of FSH and LH from the pituitary. A GnRH antagonist is administered either by injection into the muscle, or by a spray into the nostril.

On the other hand, a GnRH agonist is a mimic and initially acts like natural GnRH. It binds to the GnRH receptor on the pituitary and in so doing keeps natural GnRH from the receptors, essentially down-regulating GnRH, whilst it stimulates the secretion of FSH and LH, raising levels of these hormones in the blood. The secretion of FSH and LH causes a drop in the amount of oestrogen being produced. During this period, blood levels of FSH and LH remain high whilst oestrogen secretion is inhibited by the elevation of these hormones. After a few days the pituitary is drained of FSH and LH, and a sharp drop in the blood levels of FSH and LH occur.

The use of the agonist is to produce a sustained reduction ('down-regulation') in the release of biologically active LH by the pituitary and so prevent LH levels from rising insidiously during stimulation with gonadotropins, which may cause a premature LH surge. The length of time for down-regulation depends very much on the clinic and also the response of the patient. It is usual to start on cycle day 21 for seven to ten days and continue until down-regulation has been achieved, after which the menstrual bleed will start.

Side effects of this therapy include symptoms of hypogonadism such as are often experienced during menopause: hot flushes, night sweating, moodiness, nausea and headaches have been recorded.

THE LONG AND SHORT CYCLE

After 10 to 14 days, the process of down-regulation should have achieved its goal. At this point both the long and short cycle share similar strategies.

Using either a preparation of FSH derived from a natural source (such as pergonal or menupur) or an artificially created preparation of FSH, an FSH analogue (such as Gonal F or Follistim), the ovaries will be hyperstimulated to produce follicles. Administration is intramuscular and the patient will either receive injections at the clinic or will be asked to inject the FSH herself, usually into the superficial layer of her stomach.

At a point determined by the pelvic ultrasound scans, where a number of follicles have reached the right size indicating that the eggs have matured, a date for egg collection will be identified and the trigger injection will be provided. The patient will be told when to administer it, usually within two days of the last scan. Egg collection is usually scheduled into the diary two days after the trigger.

As you know, in a woman's natural cycle, ovulation is usually triggered by a surge in LH. LH has a short active life span and so it's not that reliable. Enter hCG, which is produced by the placenta during pregnancy. However, it has a very similar structure to LH, and it acts like LH when injected into a non-pregnant woman. The reason for its selection in IVF is that when injected into the body hCG lasts a lot longer than LH. This means that using hCG is more reliable and consistent and so the trigger used will most likely be a preparation of hCG, such as pregnyl or novarel.

Following egg collection, the eggs are laid with sperm in a culture media, a matrix that simulates conditions in the uterus, and placed in an incubator. The incubation period required for the development of a blastocyst is five days. The embryos are usually checked only on day three after egg collection and on day five preceding a blastocyst transfer.

FROZEN EMBRYO TRANSFER

Often, fresh embryos that have evolved after egg collection and are not chosen for the initial embryo transfer are frozen. This means that when it is not possible to use an embryo immediately, a frozen embryo transfer (FET) can be scheduled in at a more convenient time. In terms of thawing the embryo, and in terms of success rates, the freezing process now is much better than even five years ago, and the success rates significally so.

THE GENTLE APPROACH: NATURAL AND MILD CYCLES

The natural and mild cycles are relatively new treatment options, although the very first 'test tube' baby was conceived using this technique. It has been introduced by some clinics for several reasons that include cost, success rates in women who have low ovarian reserve or high FSH, and the health of both mother and child.

WHAT HAPPENS IN THE NATURAL IVF CYCLE?

The clinic follows a woman's natural cycle, and at egg collection retrieves the one egg that is normally and naturally produced. The drugs that are taken in this cycle are minimal, and ovarian stimulation is only provided in certain cases, for example, when low ovarian reserve has been identified by an anti-mullerian hormone (AMH) test.

In the majority of cases, the ovaries are not artificially stimulated in a natural IVF cycle. However, the cycle may be controlled with some preparations to prevent spontaneous ovulation. Progesterone is also used to enhance the chances of pregnancy. To ensure ovulation happens when the patient is most ready for embryo transfer, hCG will be administered to time the egg collection.

If a patient ovulates naturally then this might be a good cycle to consider. It has also been shown that older women seem to do better on this type of cycle than on either of the cycles mentioned above. This type of cycle should be considered if there is a familial history of cancer related to hormones.

DOES THE NUMBER OF EMBRYOS TRANSFERRED INCREASE THE CHANCES OF PREGNANCY?

The single greatest risk to giving birth to a healthy child is multiple pregnancy. Multiple pregnancies increase risks for both mother and children, both during the pregnancy and for the babies born, and these risks are significant. On the maternal side, the mother can expect increased chances of pregnancy-related high blood pressure, gestational diabetes, preeclampsia, miscarriage and potentially medical intervention at birth including either ventouse or forceps delivery. Whatever happens to the mother will be translated to the foetus and so maternal complications will exacerbate the problems faced by the babies.

For the gestating foetuses severe complications may arise. As with the mother, a multiple pregnancy increases the chances of premature birth, miscarriage and medical intervention at birth. In addition to the shared risks with the mother, babies born from a multiple pregnancy have increased chances of congenital abnormalities. Cerebral palsy, the congenital syndrome (now thought to be caused at birth) denoting motor disorders and physical disability, is highly associated with multiple pregnancy. Compared to single pregnancies, twins are four times more likely to have cerebral palsy, and in triplets the incidence of cerebral palsy is 18 times greater.

Fifty per cent of all twins are born prematurely, before 37 weeks. In triplets, 90 per cent are born prematurely. Compared to a single baby facing a premature birth, twins are five times more likely to die, and with triplets this number rises to nine.

Premature birth is associated with low birth weight. To health professionals, this innocuous phrase is anything but innocuous and implies maternal malnutrition and/or sickness during pregnancy, poor healthcare, poor prenatal care, premature birth, drug addiction, smoking, alcohol abuse and heart disease. Low birth weight significantly increases infant mortality. By how much is debatable, differentiated by factors such as living in a developing or developed world country and weight. The chance of survival for an infant born with a very low birth weight is dramatically reduced in comparison to an infant born with a low birth weight. In 2004 UNICEF[23] reported that infants weighing less than 2500g were 20 times more likely to die than infants heavier than 2500g. A study published in 2007 cites the risk of infant mortality due to low birth rate is up to 40 times[24] greater than babies born within normal birth weight ranges.

Electing a single embryo transfer has been shown to significantly decrease these risks.[25] However, it is true to say that the chances of pregnancy are diminished when choosing to transfer a single blastocyst embryo, but when a multiple embryo transfer is compared to increased cycles of single embryo transfers, the difference is negligible.[26]

Clinics do have an elective single embryo transfer policy and figures from the HFEA show that electing a single embryo transfer has become a preference for patients having IVF. All clinics will provide advice on the risks involved and comparisons between single and double embryo transfer, and it is as well for the potential mother to be well apprised of the dangers inherent in multiple embryo transfer.

Intracytoplasmic techniques

Intracytoplasmic sperm injection

In cases of male sub-fertility, or where there is evidence that the egg inhibits sperm penetration, intracytoplasmic sperm injection (ICSI) may be used (*intra* means 'inside' or within'; *cyto* means 'cell'; *plasm* means the 'living matter of the cell'). The first baby born of a micromanipulation technique known as SUZI, which preceded ICSI, was in 1990 in Rome. A recent meta-analysis shows that using ICSI significantly increases conception.[27]

The technique requires the injection of a single sperm into the cytoplasm of the egg and is undertaken in the embryology lab using micromanipulators and microinjectors.

Many commentators have raised concerns about this technique. In natural fertility, sperm 'pepper' the plasma surface of the oolemma (the membrane) of the egg, a process called acrosome reaction. This may be a competitive endeavour by the sperm, as many Darwinists argue, or it may not be. Nevertheless, it takes about 40 sperm to weaken the external layer of the oolemma before a sperm can penetrate to the cytoplasm. Immediately after penetration the oolemma hardens again and blocks any further penetration by any other sperm.

This process of acrosome reaction is entirely bypassed by ICSI and there has been quite a debate about its use. Essentially, increased levels of birth defects have been found in babies born from IVF compared with natural conception. The debate questions whether this increase is due to the treatment of infertility, or whether it is due to the aetiology of infertility itself, that is, the sperm, the reason for using ICSI in the first place. Or both. The results of a large study conducted in Australia suggest that both are causative factors. However, when a range of factors are excluded, such as age of the mother and smoking, then the authors found no significant difference between levels of birth defects in children born from IVF or from natural conception, but when IVF is combined with ICSI, then the chances of a birth defect are increased.[28] This study follows quite a few other studies evaluating the effect of ICSI, some studies showing no difference between IVF and natural conception, whilst others have arrived at the same conclusion as the Australian study. It has to be said that at this time, the jury is still out and guidance remains the same.

The Australian study is not the only study, however. In the recent past there have been quite a few, some studies showing no difference whilst others find, again, that ICSI may be the adjunctive treatment that causes increased birth defects. However, at this time, whilst the jury may still be out, it seems that ICSI may have had its day.

Gamete intrafallopian transfer

There are other techniques that have been or are being slowly pushed to the long grass. These include gamete intrafallopian transfer (GIFT) where eggs are removed from the ovary and replaced in the fallopian tube along with the sperm. This is obviously not an IVF technique since fertilisation takes place within the woman, and so replicates some of the processes of natural conception. Even though approximately 25 to 30 per cent of GIFT cycles achieve a viable pregnancy, figures that are similar to IVF figures, the technological advances in IVF make GIFT redundant in many ways, not least because IVF requires fewer surgical procedures.

Zygote intrafallopian transfer

Zygote intrafallopian transfer (ZIFT) is very similar to GIFT, and is in fact derived from that technique. Like GIFT and IVF, eggs are collected from the ovaries. Unlike GIFT and like IVF, the eggs are fertilised in vitro. Unlike both GIFT and IVF, however, the resulting embryo is quickly returned to the fallopian tube earlier than anything seen in IVF and therefore more closely replicates the natural process of conception. Like GIFT though, this technique requires more surgical procedures than IVF, and increasingly sophisticated IVF makes ZIFT less attractive.

In comparison to IVF, very few cycles of GIFT or ZIFT are now undertaken.

Assisted hatching

Assisted hatching is a technology that aids embryo implantation. In order to position and adhere to the endometrium, the zona pellucia (the membrane surrounding the embryo) must rupture. The technique was pioneered in 1990. In some cases, the zona pellucida of embryos derived from IVF may be thicker, and therefore might inhibit rupture and subsequent implantation. The pioneer of the technology, Jacques Cohen developed a method to pierce the membrane, thereby assisting with the hatching of the embryo.

When it was initiated, assisted hatching initially seemed to offer improved implantation rates, and a 2011 meta-analysis appeared to confirm that in frozen embryo transfers, assisted hatching could improve the rates of implantation and live birth.[29] More recently, however, guidelines from NICE states that 'assisted hatching is not recommended because it does not improve pregnancy rates'.[30]

4

Understanding IVF Part 2

Autologous endometrial coculture

Developed in 2004, autologous endometrial coculture is a relatively new technique, which seems to promise significant increases in pregnancy for poor responders. It is a treatment that has been shown to improve the chances for patients with repeated IVF failed cycles, and for women who unfortunately produce poor quality eggs.

Prior to an IVF cycle, the patient will have an endometrial biopsy, where a small amount of endometrial tissue is removed and sent to a lab for treatment and freezing. The patient undergoes a normal IVF cycle, has egg collection, and the eggs are fertilised with sperm. At this point the layer of endometrium that was removed and frozen prior to the IVF cycle is thawed and grown. When embryos evolve, they are laid on top of the thawed endometrium and over the next few days are watched for development. If development has occurred and the embryos are healthy, they are then transferred to the uterus.

Evidence suggests that this process is much more successful for patients who have poor quality eggs, or have suffered repeated IVF failures, than transferring egg and sperm into the culture media as per the normal IVF cycle.[1, 2]

Embryo splitting and cloning

The creation of identical embryos occurs naturally when the zygote splits spontaneously. The process has been replicated artificially and employed in labs on animals since the 1980s. In animals, the technology often used is called nuclear transfer and involves transferring the genetic material of one egg to a cell that has been enucleated, that is, has had its genetic material removed. However, embryo splitting is also used in animals for genotyping, hereditary diseases and sex determination.[3, 4, 5]

Embryo splitting in human embryos was first undertaken by researchers at George Washington University in the early 1990s. It is also known as cloning.

Embryos are essentially pluripotent cells. The term 'pluripotent' is one of several used to classify the differentiability of stem cells:

1. The term 'totipotent' reflects the potential of this class of cell. Totipotency refers to stem cells with the ability to differentiate into an entirely new and viable organism. Although not synonymous, it is reasonable to think of omnipotent when thinking of totipotent. In an embryo, totipotent cells are the first cells to divide.

2. Pluripotency refers to cells that are able to differentiate into any of the tissues arising from the three essential germ layers present in homo sapiens (mesoderms), so pluripotent cells cannot give rise to a viable organism, but can differentiate into any tissue.

3. Multipotency refers to stem cells that are less potent but can differentiate into cells that are from a similar origin. For example, lymphocytes are of haematopoietic origin. A multipotent haematopoietic stem cell can differentiate into a lymphocyte but not into osteoblasts.

4. Oligopotency refers to cells that are capable of differentiating into a few cell types.

5. Unipotency refers to cells that can differentiate into one cell type only. This type of cell is often referred to as precursor.

Embryo splitting involves the division of a two-cell, four-cell, or eight-cell embryo. Since a two-cell embryo can be split and develop into two genetically identical embryos, it is possible that a four-cell embryo would create four new, genetically identical embryos and similarly, splitting an eight-cell embryo could result in eight genetically identical embryos.

Researchers at George Washington studied the technology on human embryos.[6] The technique they used involved dissolving the zona pelludica of the embryo, then coating each individual cell with an artificial zona pellucida, which allowed the cell to continue to evolve. Since the cell was totipotent it could evolve into a viable embryo and after implantation, a viable foetus.

At this time, the technology is used mainly in the farming industry. But how close is the use of this technique in human IVF? What would be the reasons for its inclusion in current IVF procedures? Would we want such a technique to be made available? Would you want to use it?

This technique was pioneered in the early 1990s. The National Human Genome Research Institute identifies three different types of cloning technology: gene cloning, which clones DNA for research purposes; reproductive cloning, which creates copies of animals; and therapeutic cloning, which creates embryonic stem cells to research the potential to grow replacement tissue.[7]

When applied to animals, the technology offers the possibility of transgenetics, a potential already fulfilled to some extent. Polly, the first transgenic sheep, expressed one of the essential therapeutics for haemophiliacs, clotting factor IX, in her milk once she had matured. Other potentials are envisioned: nucleating cells in animals with our own DNA to grow specific tissue types, for instance, would have an extraordinary impact for transplant patients, since the tissue type grown would be exactly the same as the DNA donor and therefore potential organ rejection could be avoided. Another example would be genetically modifying pancreatic islets to secrete insulin once transplanted into the DNA donor. Or, to follow the example of Polly, the milk we drink in the future might come from genetically modified animals that produce milk with specific health-enhancing proteins, or antibodies or to reduce the effects of dementia.

In 2008 the US Food and Drug Administration (FDA) published a report that food derived from cloned animals was as safe to eat as any other food we eat every day and could be included in the human food chain.[8]

A report published in 1993 discusses the possibilities inherent in this technology, and why it may be of benefit to infertile or sub-fertile patients.[9] First, splitting an embryo could potentially reduce the number of IVF cycles a woman might require. She would only have to go through one cycle of IVF, only have to have her ovaries hyperstimulated once, only have to suffer the potential risks of an IVF cycle once, and possibly have eight viable embryos from one embryo. Second, if a woman suffers the loss of her ovaries, for instance from chemotherapy, embryos could be created prior to the chemotherapy. Those might be the last chance she has to become pregnant. To be able to create eight embryos from a single embryo would significantly increase her chances to reproduce later in life.

Embryo splitting also increases the possibility that a couple might be able to exclude hereditary disease by increasing the number of embryos available for pre-implantation genetic diagnosis (PGD) (see Chapter 5).

Although fertility clinics are able to determine the sex of the child, it is illegal to do so in the UK unless the parent has a serious genetic condition. The technology to do this is PGD.

Risks

Cancer

The circulating steroid hormone oestrogen is a natural part of a woman's reproductive life. In addition to its other functions, such as cholesterol management, it stimulates cell production in breast, endometrial and uterine tissues every menstrual cycle.

Epidemiological studies have shown a strong correlation between oestrogen and cancer, particularly breast, endometrial and uterine cancers. Women who begin menstruating early or have a late menopause have a higher risk of breast cancer, and oestrogen is the prime suspect. The reason that oestrogen has been thought to be carcinogenic is because of its actions on cells. Oestrogen binds to receptors in cells and in so doing activates genes which cause the cells to produce more cells, an action called cell proliferation. If one of these cells has mutations that are potentially carcinogenic, then the action of oestrogen will cause that cell to divide and produce more cells like it. In contradistinction to oestrogen, progesterone appears to protect the woman against ovarian cancer.[10]

'Oestrogen' is actually a collective noun; there are several forms of oestrogen, and not all of them increase the risk of cancer.[11] However, the fact that oestrogen induces cell proliferation should mean that all oestrogens are carcinogenic, and the fact that not all oestrogens are carcinogenic creates a dichotomy.

An influential study published in 2003 has shown that there are actually two pathways by which oestrogen may cause cancer, the second involving a process called oxidative stress.[12]

Reactive oxygen species (ROS) are necessary for the normal functioning of the human body, but when they are out of balance, as when oxidative stress occurs, they can be dangerous, causing harm to many cellular functions and many molecules necessary for healthy functioning. Oxidative stress is implicated in many conditions including hypertension, diabetes and Parkinson's disease. It also damages DNA.

Since oxidative stress can cause damage in the brain and thereby impair healthy functioning of the nervous system, it is unsurprising that oxidative stress has now been associated with anxiety, emotional and psychological stress both as a causal factor and as a factor caused by these conditions.[13, 14]

The 2003 study evaluated the effect of the known carcinogenic oestrogen, 17beta-estradiol (E2). E2 causes cell proliferation, as per the theory, and when it is metabolised by the cell causes oxygen radicals to be produced. In the study, the researchers also evaluated the effect of a non-carcinogenic oestrogen, an oestrogen that is not easily metabolised by a cell and so, following the theory, oxygen radicals should be produced. However, when oxygen radicals were added to the non-carcinogenic oestrogen, cancer occurred. The authors concluded that (a) the second pathway in oestrogen carcinogenesis relies, at least in part, on oxidative stress, (b) that because 17beta-estradiol causes cell proliferation and oxidative stress, its potential as a carcinogen is very high and (c) even non-carcinogenic oestrogens may become carcinogenic in the presence of oxidative stress. As a result of this study, oestrogen has now been added to the watch list of carcinogens maintained by the National Institute of Environmental Health Sciences in the US.

There is a correlation between the amount of oestrogen a woman is exposed to and breast cancer. More oestrogen, and more oestrogen over a longer period of time, generally puts a patient at a greater risk. There is also now an association between oxidative stress and oestrogenic carcinogenesis, and an association between oxidative stress and emotional and psychological stress. It is from this perspective that it is important to consider the effect of IVF on a woman's health.

In contradistinction to oestrogen, progesterone appears to protect women against ovarian cancer.[15]

BREAST CANCER

Some studies have found an association between IVF hormone preparations and breast cancer, and particularly for women older than 40, whilst other research has found none, and so the matter remains controversial. If the associations are found to be true, however, the numbers are very small and the risk still appears to be low.[16, 17, 18]

OVARIAN CANCER

During her life, there is a small but persistent chance that a woman may develop ovarian cancer (1.8%). The causes are thought to be chemical carcinogens processed locally, repeated ovulations, and stimulation of the hormones FSH and LH by their action on oestrogen, or by their action on the ovaries. Breastfeeding and lactation, early menopause and oral contraceptives seem to reduce the chance of developing this form of cancer. The incidence of ovarian cancer is slightly increased in women with sub-fertility problems.

Since the late 1980s, however, researchers have investigated whether treatment for fertility using gonadotropins for stimulation of the ovaries and/or inducing ovulation increases the chance of ovarian cancer. Since the publication of the first research trial showing an association between fertility treatment and ovarian cancer,[19] trials investigating this association have progressively become larger and more sophisticated.

In 1992, a study published findings that women who had taken fertility drugs were 2.7 times more likely to develop ovarian cancer than women who had not.[20] This meant that almost 4 per cent of women who underwent IVF treatment were likely to develop ovarian cancer. However, the authors also showed that women who did become pregnant through IVF didn't develop ovarian cancer, suggesting that it may be the fertility problem that caused the cancer, and that IVF treatment might exacerbate that problem.

This study, by Whittermore and colleagues, has been criticised on a number of levels, not least for the lack of definition of the substances referred to as 'fertility medications', why they were taken, or the doses and frequency of administration. The study was also small. On the other hand, Rossing *et al.* found a significantly increased risk of ovarian cancer in women who had taken clomiphene over a long time. In this study, ranging from 1974–1985, 11 cases of ovarian tumours were found in a cohort of 3,837 infertile women, of which five tumours were borderline. The authors found that in comparison to infertile women who did not take clomiphene citrate, infertile women who *did* take clomiphene citrate were more at risk of developing ovarian tumour (borderline or not), and that risk was elevated in women who used clomiphene citrate for more than 12 IVF cycles.[21]

In 1999 *The Lancet* published a study by Venn *et al.* who investigated a population of 30,000 women and found no incidence of association in either breast or ovarian cancer in women having IVF treatment, but they did find an association of ovarian cancer in women who were diagnosed with unexplained infertility.[22] This study was confirmed in 2002 in the Ness analysis of eight research studies, a population of 13,000 women.[23] The conclusion of Ness was that infertility alone, and not the treatment of infertility, caused ovarian cancer.

More recently, other large analyses have provided more data. In 2011 researchers led by Professor van Leeuwen from the Netherlands Cancer Institute evaluated the long-term effects of IVF treatment over 15 years. This study found that compared to the 6006 women who were having difficulty conceiving and did not receive IVF treatment, the 19,146 women who did have IVF treatment were four times more likely to develop borderline ovarian tumours, that is, not life-threatening ovarian cancer.[24] In contrast, research published in 2013 comparing the records of 20,000 women who did not receive IVF treatment against 67,000 women who did concluded that, although some instances of ovarian and breast cancer did occur, the numbers were so small they were statistically insignificant.[25]

Birth defects

There has been research published over the last few years showing that IVF significantly increases the chance of birth defects. There has also been research that disputes those findings. A study from 2004 showed that 8.6 per cent of children born from IVF, and 9 per cent of children born from IVF + ICSI, were diagnosed with a major birth defect by age one. This compares with 4.2 per cent of children born from natural conception.[26]

In 2006 a study from Denmark found that there was a slightly higher risk of defects in children born from infertile patients who conceived naturally compared to fertile parents.[27] At the same time but in the US, scientists from UCLA looked at babies born between 2006 and 2007 and discriminated between babies born as a result of IVF (4795) and babies born from natural fertility (46,025) but who had similar maternal demographics. In total, 3463 babies were born with major birth defects but birth defects were significantly increased for babies born after IVF (9%) compared with naturally conceived babies (6.6%). The scientists reported that the odds are 1.25 times greater for potential defects in babies born as a result of IVF than naturally conceived babies. In France, researchers evaluated 15,000 babies born from IVF treatments and found the risk of congenital abnormalities doubled as a result of IVF treatments in comparison to babies born from natural conception.[28]

Interestingly, a study from 1999 reported that ovarian hyperstimulation has a negative effect on implantation which appears to be due to endometrial receptivity.[29] The investigators found that by decreasing the dose of gonadotropins to produce a mild stimulation of the ovaries, increased embryo implantation was significantly increased in patients receiving a low-dose IVF protocol in comparison to patients receiving the dose in standard IVF.

Low-dose IVF also appears to influence birth weight. In research published in the European Journal of Obstetrics and Gynecology, patients who selected the natural-cycle IVF protocol gave birth to babies that were, on average, 134g heavier than those conceived from standard IVF regimens.[30] A higher birth weight indicates better gestation and better prospects for the baby. Mild IVF is less expensive than standard IVF, since the hormones and drugs are reduced, and more comfortable for patients, since the number of visits and the number of injections are reduced. The side effects are also reduced and there are fewer multiple births. In terms of cost, comfort and quality, mild, low-dose or even natural IVF appear attractive alternatives to patients seeking help and treatment for infertility.

5

Western Conventional Medicine

An Integrated Diagnosis

Introduction

Most couples are fertile, although the number of fertile couples appears to be diminishing. Statistically, most couples (84%) will conceive naturally within a year of having regular sex without contraception, and 92 per cent will conceive after two years.[1] Regular sex is defined as every two to three days. If this has been the case and the patient has not conceived, then investigations are called for.

Fertility is limited by age, the presence and extent of conditions outlined below and factors that are currently inexplicable. Of course, every person is unique, as is every couple. I have met couples who have suffered several IVF failures only to get pregnant naturally and I have met seemingly fertile couples who, even with many investigations, have required assisted reproductive techniques.

Investigations should be undertaken earlier if there is a known cause or if the couple think that there might be a potential cause for concern. In the UK, the National Health Service advise that if a woman is over 35 she should seek further investigations within a year of trying to conceive.[2] However, in my view, if the couple are nearing 30 and have been trying for six months, why wait? There might be a very simple cause inhibiting or obstructing conception that might require medical attention or makes pregnancy impossible without IVF. Once the decision has been made to have children, it seems more sensible to seek investigations as early as possible.

What to include in a diagnosis

An integrated diagnosis will include both traditional medical (TM) and Western medical (WM) categories. Whereas WM colleagues may not derive much from TM terms, traditional medical pracitioners can derive a lot from WM diagnostic terms and investigations. Such a diagnosis may take some time.

A full description of the main complaint is required in both TM and WM terms. The diagnosis will look at a patient's personal history: age, children, any complications during previous pregnancies and/or birth, miscarriages, length of time since contraception was stopped, length of time trying to conceive. It's also important to discuss sexual intercourse.

The physiological history should consider a systems review, family history, a gynaecological review and a review of any medication, current or past. It's also useful to include a general checklist of the patient's past examinations, internal investigations and bloods, and a gynaecological/fertility checklist of examinations. The review should also include the body mass index (BMI) and the waist to hip ratio (WHR).

The body mass index

The body mass index (BMI) was devised by the Belgian polymath, Adolphe Quetelet in the middle of the nineteeth century. The measure is worked out by dividing the mass of the individual by the square of their height and is usually expressed as kg/m^2.

$$BMI = mass\ (kg)/[height\ (m)]^2$$

The BMI provides the following indications:

- underweight = <18.5
- normal weight = 18.5–24.9
- overweight = 25–29.9
- obesity = 30 or greater
- morbid obesity = 40 or greater.

The BMI was originally devised to identify how sedentary a person is. Since that time the World Health Organization has developed a useful chart indicating BMI correlation with obesity.[3] A healthy BMI lies within the range 18.5–25. The upper limit of this range was adopted by the US in 1998 when the National Institutes of Health reduced the upper level from BMI 27.8 to 25, and at a stroke increased the population of unhealthy Americans by more than 10 per cent.

To give you an idea of just how worrisome the level of obesity is, in 1994 more than half the US population had a BMI over 25, and roughly 3 per cent of those had a BMI of more than 40, that is, were morbidly obese. Figures published by the Information service for the National Institute of Diabetes and Digestive and Kidney Diseases (NIDDK) in 2013 for the years 2009–2010 show that more than two-thirds (68.8%) of Americans older than 20 years of age are either overweight or obese; more than 35 per cent of American adults are obese and more than 6 per cent of American adults are extremely obese.[4]

In England, more people are overweight or obese than not.[5] Reports show levels of obesity are rising and causation does not appear to be related to income differences, social class or gender.[6] Reporting on the levels of obesity in the UK, the Health and Social Care Information Centre (HSCIC) state that in England, just over 40 per cent of women had a BMI within normal range in comparison to 32 per cent of men; conversely, 32 per cent of women and 42 per cent of men were overweight. Almost a quarter of the population (25 per cent) were obese. The HSCIC also provide a progressive trend in obesity from 1993 to 2012; in the male population obesity rose from 13.2 per cent in 1993 to 24.4 per cent in 2012, and in the female population obesity rose from 16.4 per cent in 1993 to 25.1 per cent in 2012.[7]

That 25 per cent of the population in England is obese is shocking. However, the HSCIC document makes reference to a 2007 report provided by the Government Office for Science predicting that in ten years' time 36 per cent of the female population will be obese. In men it's predicted to double: by 2025, nearly 50 per cent of the male population will be obese.[8]

Waist to hip ratio

BMI is a useful indicator of lifestyle and future problems. However, the waist to hip ratio (WHR) appears to provide a clearer picture of health and fertility.[9] The WHR is the ratio of the circumference of the waist to the hips.[10] For women, a WHR of 0.7 is ideal. There is evidence that shows that women with a WHR of 0.8 have a significantly reduced chance of getting pregnant.[11]

The formula is:

WHR = waist/hip

The WHO suggests that the waist circumference should be measured midway between the lower rib and the top of the hip (crest of the iliac) – about 2.5cm above the tummy button, at the level of Shuifen, Ren 9, and the hip measurement should be taken around the widest area of the buttocks. The tape should be parallel to the floor.

Lifestyle

Many mothers-to-be are employed. It's useful to determine the stress levels she might be enduring: the type of employment she has, how often she works, the number of hours she works and what other work she is doing outside her main employment will give an indication.

Other areas that should be discussed include any history of smoking, alcohol consumption, and/or any other drugs (including so-called 'recreational' drugs); diet (omnivore or not), number of meals per day, weekly intake of meat, vegetables, fruit, chocolate, fizzy drinks, tea and coffee, and sugar.

Exercise

Exercise is important, not just for fertility but also for life. Exercise provides obvious health benefits across most major biological systems and causes the secretion of endorphins, which improve mood, reduce stress, increase self-esteem and help with sleep. Exercise is an effective self-help treatment for mild to moderate depression and also reduces anxiety. This latter point is very important when it comes to fertility-related stress.

Fortunately, many women are aware of this, and are taking classes or including exercise in their daily lives. Guidelines in the UK for a healthy adult life provide that we should be doing at least two and a half hours of medium to intense aerobic exercise per week, and muscle building activities on two or more days per week. Aerobic activity can be fast walking, dancing, hiking or cycling, or a game of doubles tennis or volleyball every week. Alternatively, 75 minutes of vigorous activity is equivalent to two and a half hours of moderate intense aerobic exercise and includes activities such as jogging, singles tennis or aerobics. In terms of muscle work, anything that uses body weight as resistance, such as yoga or push-ups or sits, is good. Weight training is also very popular. However, too much of a good thing can be bad and too much intense exercise can affect reproductivity.

* * *

It is estimated that 20–30 per cent of cases of sub-fertility in women are diagnosed as unexplained. There are many factors involved.

The uterus

Traditional Chinese medicine understands the central aspects of reproduction as balanced correspondence between the Heart, Uterus and Kidneys. The Heart and Uterus communicate via the Uterus Vessel (the Bao Mai); the Kidneys and the Uterus communicate via the Uterus Channel (the Bao Luo). The Uterus itself was not differentiated into its substructures but also embraced the fallopian tubes, the cervix, and the ovaries (the Bao Gong). Functionally it is comprised of both yin and yang aspects; discharging and holding.

In some cases, the uterus may have developed in such a way that natural conception is either inhibited or made impossible. In the very rare condition of agenesis, the vagina does not form properly and the uterus either does not form at all or is very small. This condition makes conception very difficult indeed, if not impossible. In other uterine abnormalities, natural conception and pregnancy is still possible but made more of a journey. Carrying the baby to term is the key factor here.

Uterine abnormalities

Uterus didelphys, where the uterus has two cavities and each cavity may lead to its own cervix and vagina, does not affect the ability to carry a baby to term, although the matter of twins will need discussion.

The unicornuate uterus has only one horn, in comparison to a normal uterus. Although a woman may have two ovaries, only one will be actively involved in reproduction, since the single horn will be related to only one ovary.

The bicornuate uterus is similar to the septate uterus. The top of the uterus, the fundus, extends deep in to the uterine cavity, almost bisecting the uterus, giving an image of two horns. In this condition, pregnancy is still possible but miscarriages are far more common and a lot of support will be necessary.

The septate uterus, like the bicornuate uterus, may be significantly or partially bisected. However, the impediment is not the fundus but a fibrous tissue, the septum, which extends down from the fundus and into the uterine cavity. The size of the septum determines the chances of miscarriage. However, septate uteri do not prevent natural conception, and it's more common to have a partial septate uterus than a complete septate.

The arcuate uterus is fairly common. In this case, the fundus is slightly thicker in the middle section, and so extends slightly into the uterine cavity. It usually has very little impact on pregnancy or live birth.

DIAGNOSIS OF UTERINE ABNORMALITIES

In all except the agenesis uterine abnormality, where diagnosis will arise in early adulthood, the diagnosis of uterine abnormalities will occur when a patient is having trouble conceiving or is having difficulty carrying a baby to term. Diagnosis can be fairly straightforward; ultrasound may be suggested, or magnetic resonance imaging (MRI). Otherwise a hystero contrast sonography (HyCoSy) or laparoscopy may be advised. It's probably useful to determine the shape of the uterus early in the fertility journey to avoid the potential distress of miscarriage.

Cervical mucus

The role of cervical mucus is to help the passage of sperms by protecting them from the slightly acidic nature of the vagina, and to provide nourishment for the sperm's journey to the fallopian tubes. In good cervical mucus, sperm can last up to 72 hours within the uterus. The mucus itself undergoes several morphological changes in response to increases in oestrogen. In the lead up to ovulation, the mucus can be fairly thick and slightly white. As oestrogen increases, so the mucus becomes thinner and clearer, more like egg white, until ovulation. It is possible to test the nature of the mucus by stretching it between the thumb and forefinger. The stretchier it is, the better. Within 24 hours of ovulation the mucus changes again and forms a thick plug in the cervix.

The nature and quality of cervical mucus is very important in natural fertility. As the follicular phase advances, both quantity and quality of cervical mucus should increase under the influence of oestrogen. As cervical mucus becomes more oestrogenic (stretchier, clearer), it becomes more alkaline and secretes down the vaginal canal. The point of ovulation is the most fertile moment, when the cervical mucus should be most alkaline. Sperm can survive in an alkaline environment of pH7.2–7.8. After ovulation the cervical mucus changes nature again.

In some cases, cervical mucus may not be present, or be present in such small amounts that it does not contribute to the sperm's journey. In other cases cervical mucus may become hostile.

There are four categories of hostile cervical mucus: it may become thick and prevent the passage of sperm; it may produce anti-sperm antibodies that disrupt the motile (swimming) nature of sperm; it may become acidic in nature – sperm are comfortable in an alkaline solution (pH7.2–7.8); in an acidic environment (the natural vaginal environment is pH3–4), sperm will not survive long. Both cervical mucus and vaginal pH are defence mechanisms in general, but change during the menstrual cycle. Finally, inflammatory cells in the mucus may arise from an infection – the cells will react to the sperm as foreign bodies and consume them.

Diagnosis of cervical mucus can initially be undertaken by the patient, using the finger stretch test. If the cervical mucus remains thick, or if there is very little of it, then dietary and fluid advice should be given – drinking more water and less coffee/tea or fizzy drinks can make a difference. Chinese herbal medicine can also improve mucosal quality.[15] In the event that increased mucosal quality still makes no difference, it is advisable to seek further tests.

Fibroids

Uterine fibroids, also called fibromyomas, leiomyomas or myomas, are benign, non-cancerous fibrous tissue masses (also called tumours) that grow in the uterus or around the uterus. They vary in size; some are relatively small whilst others can become quite large. From a WM perspective the cause of their growth is unexplained, although oestrogen is sometimes implicated since size sometimes fluctuates according to oestrogen levels: when oestrogen levels are elevated, the size of a fibroid may increase. Often, fibroids are asymptomatic and do not influence potential pregnancy at all. In other cases, fibroids can and do.

Size does matter. Fibroids can be very small whilst others can be the size of a football. The larger a fibroid grows, however, the more likely it will influence blood flow in the pelvic area. If a fibroid grows very large it can press on other organs and affect other systems. There may not be a direct effect on fertility per se, but the structures that support a pregnancy may well be influenced.

The fibroids that concern us most are those that directly interfere with uterine function. Of the five main fibroid categories, both intramural fibroids and sub-mucosal fibroids grow into the uterus and are therefore likely to affect fertility. Cervical fibroids may also influence fertility, for obvious reasons. Both subserosal and pedunculated fibroids grow outside the uterus and penetrate into the pelvis. These fibroids can grow very large.

SYMPTOMS

Whilst fibroids can be small and asymptomatic (bearing in mind that being small and asymptomatic may not go hand in hand), symptoms can and do occur. The menstrual period can become prolonged. Other symptoms may include frequent urination or difficulty with urination, backache that may refer down the legs, pressure or pain in the pelvic area and constipation. In both intramural and submucosal fibroids, the menstrual bleed can be very heavy and can even become dangerous, leading to anaemia and even low blood count. Diagnosis relies on ultrasound, MRI, HyCoSy or laparoscopy.

TREATMENTS

Where the fibroids are small, treatment may not be required. It is only where the growth interferes with natural processes that medical intervention is advised; fertility patients will be advised by their clinic.

Fallopian tube damage

Fallopian tubes actively contribute to the journey of the egg and, where fertilisation has occurred, the journey of the embryo to the uterus. In addition to smooth muscle contraction, microscopic ciliated cells, like hairs, line the inner surface of the fallopian tube. At ovulation, the cilia move in a synchronous beat and egg transport appears to rely on the synchronous beat frequency of the cilia to carry it towards the ampulla and on to the uterus. If the egg becomes fertilised, the function of the cilia continues uninterrupted, carrying the embryo to the uterus.

The functions of the fallopian tubes may become impaired by various factors, both extrinsic and intrinsic, including environmental factors such as smoking that may damage these delicate structures.[12, 13] Absolute cessation of ciliary movement, known as Kartagener's Syndrome, or primary ciliary dyskinesia, is also associated with sub-fertility.

The fallopian tubes may become damaged. This may be a result of chlamydia, the silent sexually transmitted disease, or surgery or endometriosis, causing tubal occlusion. Blocked tubes will render a woman infertile and she will require IVF. If a single tube is blocked then a woman's chances of becoming pregnant will be halved when both ovaries are functioning normally. If the tube is damaged but still functional, its ability to transport the egg may still be possible if not entirely impaired. However, where damage has occurred, the cilia or the ciliary beat frequency, or fallopian tube contractility may become impaired. Similarly, if the uterus has suffered scarring then implantation may also become impaired but for exceptional circumstances, such as the uterine scratch.[14]

Ovulatory problems

In the main, ovulation disorders are caused by PCOS, thyroid problems including overactive thyroid (hyperthyroidism) and underactive thyroid (hypothyroidism), and premature ovarian failure (POF).

WAYS TO IDENTIFY OVULATION

The only true test for ovulation is pregnancy. However, ultrasound provides a very strong indication of ovulation. There are many good ovulation kits on the market that will give a good indication whether the patient has ovulated or not. Ovulation detection can be significantly augmented if the patient starts and maintains a BBT. This will also help in the diagnosis of the patient and if the patient isn't imminently embarking on an IVF cycle, starting a BBT should be encouraged.

Polycystic ovarian syndrome

Polycystic ovaries have many cysts, unruptured follicles that are less than 8mm. The presence of the cysts is a reflection of ovarian dysfunction and a cycle that inhibits further growth and rupture of follicles. The problem of 'polycystic ovaries', where the ovaries have a large number of cysts, is not to be confused with polycystic ovarian syndrome (PCOS). Polycystic ovarian syndrome affects around 20 per cent of women in their reproductive years.

A syndrome is not a disease, but a group of symptoms. When a symptom is identified, the clinician is alerted to the possibility that more symptoms associated with the syndrome will possibly occur. The symptoms associated with PCOS include an irregular menstrual cycle, or no menstrual cycle at all; sub-fertility and anovulation; hirsutism, where certain male traits occur such as hair growth on the face, chest, legs and back; hair loss on the head; weight gain and obesity; oily skin and acne. Hormone levels of oestrogen, testosterone, AMH and insulin are higher than normal. Later in life, PCOS is associated with higher cholesterol levels and type 2 diabetes.

The cause of PCOS is unexplained in WM. However, there is evidence that it may have a genetic component.[16] In fact, there are suggestions that PCOS may be a survival trait in homo sapiens. Some literature also implicates xenoestrogens of artificial origin and obesity. The pathogenesis of the syndrome involves the inhibition of natural ovulation, and subsequent ovarian stimulation of oestrogen and androgens (male hormones). Although elevated androgens can be a result of excessive LH secretion dysregulated at the hypothalamic level causing inappropriate GNrH secretion, elevated androgens are also thought to be the cause of increased LH secretion. This is a vicious circle, exacerbated by excess oestrogen-reducing FSH secretion, leading to a decline in ovarian function to transform androgens to oestrogen.

Adipose tissue has endocrinological properties: it secretes oestrogens, androgens and leptin. Elevated insulin may be a result of insulin resistance (hyperinsulinemia) and/or increased body weight. Although leptin has been shown to potentiate the effect of elevated insulin levels on GnrH secretion it has no effect on its own.[17]

Hyperinsulinemia is quite common in normal as well as overweight patients and induces increased GnRH pulse frequency from the hypothalamus, which naturally elevates LH secretion and reduces FSH secretion.

WM treatment of PCOS involves laparoscopic ovarian drilling (LOD) to excise androgenic tissue in the ovaries, stimulating the menstrual cycle by stimulating ovulation, or reducing the vicious circle by attempting to rectify androgenism with cyclic application of progesterone.

ADJUNCTIVE TREATMENTS FOR PCOS

Self-help

Body weight is very important. Diet, insulin resistance and increased body weight/obesity are common factors in PCOS. Which causes the other is a matter of debate. Insulin resistance (IR) is caused by high levels of insulin secreted over a long time (i.e. years). Dense, high-energy foods elevate insulin secretion. A diet of dense, high-energy foods elevates insulin secretion and over a long time and can lead to IR. Moreover, although animal studies have shown a high fat diet significantly increases insulin resistance in a very short time,[18] implying that diet is the primary cause, and insulin resistance in humans is correlated with a high fat/low fibre diet.[19] Because the function of insulin (to deliver glucose to the muscles) is impaired, IR increases appetite. IR is a precursor to diabetes.

Increased body weight derived from an increased sugar/high fat diet is also associated with leptin resistance, meaning that, although there may be elevated plasma leptin levels, the hypothalamus still recognises an energy deficient state and stimulates feeding. As a result, weigh increases.

In addition to long-term health issues, adipose tissue secretes oestrogen and androgens and as a result potentially inhibits reasonable correspondence within the HPO axis. Adipose tissue also secretes leptin; leptin modulates insulin and so adipose tissue modulates blood sugar levels. An initial treatment plan should include patient support in weight management, to establish and maintain a *living* exercise and diet plan, for example, to reduce the amount of adipose tissue.

Living, here, refers to the manner in which a woman engages with the process, where exercise and diet plans are more than just products that one might purchase and then dispose of once used, but are maintained and become deeply embedded in one's life. More often than not, IVF is a hard and demanding journey, and many changes in a woman's life are required during that journey; taking charge of the changes that are required to facilitate and augment potential success can lead to the development of habits that are beneficial and life enhancing. If these positive habits are 'lived' they will be embedded and will become part of a woman's everyday life. What I am aiming for is for a woman to have acquired value from the journey, whatever its outcome. It's ambitious, but, having established these plans with patients I have seen long-term beneficial lifestyle changes as a result of the IVF journey.

Acupuncture

Research has been undertaken in the West to investigate the effect of acupuncture on PCOS. A review undertaken in Australia[20] evaluated all trials published in English and on humans between 1970 and 2009. Although the number of studies included was relatively small, this review concluded that, in addition to being a safe and effective treatment for PCOS, acupuncture treatments in the treatment of PCOS have a range of beneficial effects including the increase of blood flow to the ovaries, increasing insulin sensitivity and decreasing blood glucose and insulin levels, reducing cortisol levels and assisting in weight loss.

A more recent randomised controlled trial from Sweden showed that acupuncture and exercise reduced circulating androgens, reduced acne and improved menstrual frequency. The authors concluded that the effect of low-frequency electro-acupuncture was superior to physical exercise and may have a role to play in the treatment of hyperandrogensim and oligo/amenorrhea.[21]

Chinese herbal medicine

In terms of Chinese herbal medicine (CHM), a recent Cochrane review found that improved clinical pregnancy outcomes are associated with the combination therapy of CHM and clomiphene.[22] However, the authors also point out that evidence is limited by the number and quality of the trials.

Endometriosis

Endometriosis is a common, chronic ailment. In the UK it's estimated that two million women between the ages of 25 and 40 are affected by this condition. The condition involves endometrial cells or fragments of endometrial tissue adhering to tissue outside of the uterus.

CAUSES OF ENDOMETRIOSIS

It is not known how endometrial cells or fragments of endometria escape the uterus other than during normal menstruation. A popular theory is that, instead of being discharged in the normal menstrual bleed, the endometrial cells travel in the opposite direction and exit the uterus through the fallopian tubes. Once outside the uterus the cells adhere to secondary tissue. Adhesions can occur in the fallopian tubes or ovaries, on the bladder or bowel, vagina, rectum or even nervous tissue. There have also been reports of adhesions in the lungs and on the stomach. The secondary adhesion, called endometrial tissue implants, reacts to hormonal fluctuations in the same manner as the endometrium and fluctuates in size according to oestrogenic influence. However, in contradistinction to the endometrium, although there may be a little bleeding, the implant does not appear to shed at the end of the month.

You would think that the immune system would deal with the implant. In fact, some researchers have considered the possibility that the immune system in women with endometriosis behaves in a different way and there does seem to be an inheritable influence, since women with mothers or sisters with endometriosis also seem more likely to develop this condition.

SIGNS AND SYMPTOMS OF ENDOMETRIOSIS

Although women with superficial endometriosis may have very little pain at all, pain is a key feature of this condition. This is part of the normal physiological reaction; because the tissue reacts to the hormonal environment, when it grows and swells the inflammatory response reacts by causing the secretion of cytokines and other inflammatory signalling molecules, which is normally interpreted as pain. Pain can also be caused by the adhesions on organs that may distort or dislocate as a result of hormonal influence.

Other symptoms include heavy periods, irregular bleeding, dysmenorrhoea with pain that is cramping or sharp, or both, and can be extreme; dyspareunia (painful sex); dysuria, which may include painful urination and urgency; pain, which can be severe, in the lower abdomen, lower back or pelvis, or with bowel movements and which may refer down the legs; and sub-fertility. It may also lead to energy loss and depression.

Endometriosis is clearly related to sub-fertility, but the exact cause of this has yet to be elucidated. There are several schools of thought on what the reasons might be. Endometriosis can cause the (temporary) dislocation or distortion of organs, such as the ovaries or the fallopian tubes. The scarring from adhesions may inhibit or completely block the transit of the egg or embryo to the uterus. Such distortion/dislocation may also cause secretion of cytokines that may inhibit implantation, or may be inimical to embryo evolvement. Moreover, since prostaglandins are involved in implantation, the elevated levels of prostaglandins may interfere with that process. It may also be that endometriosis occurs in women who would have difficulty conceiving in any case.

CONVENTIONAL TREATMENTS

Painkillers, usually nonsteroidal anti-inflammatory drugs (NSAIDs) such as ibuprofen or naproxen are used to relieve the pain. If there is severe pain a combination oral contraceptive is often prescribed.

Since endometriotic implants respond to oestrogen fluctuations, GnRH analogues have been used and are effective in reducing the size and pain of implants. The downside to these drugs is that they also cause the climacteric symptoms of menopause. Symptoms can be alleviated, however, by 'add back therapy'; that is, by administering small amounts of oestrogen and progesterone.

Other drugs have also been developed, such as progestins, danazol and the experimental aromatase inhibitors, but have side effects that are more common and may prove unacceptable to the patient.

Surgery is considered the superior choice for patients undergoing fertility treatment.

Pelvic inflammatory disease

Pelvic inflammatory disease (PID) is most often seen in women under the age of 25 who are sexually active. It is caused by bacterial infection from unprotected sex leading to the transmission of a sexually transmitted infection (STI), usually gonorrhoea or chlamydia. PID can also be caused by viral, fungal or parasitic infections. Other causes of PID include intrauterine devices (IUDs), miscarriage or termination.

The inflammation eventually causes tissue damage, scarring and adhesions. Adhesions are scar tissue formations between organs and tissue. When these formations occur in the fallopian tubes they are the primary cause of sub-fertility derived from this condition.

SYMPTOMS

Symptoms include fever, lower abdominal pain, foul smelling discharge, painful sex and/or painful urination, pain in the upper right abdomen (Fitz-Hugh Curtis syndrome) and irregular periods. However, not all people experience these symptoms and often PID can be asymptomatic. In these cases, PID can still cause serious damage though. This is important because PID can be cured, but the effects of this disease are often permanent, so the sooner it is diagnosed and treated, the better. For example, PID causes scarring, which can occur within the genital system, and cause chronic pelvic pain. It can spread to the liver, causing Fitz-Hugh Curtis syndrome.

DIAGNOSIS

If PID is suspected, diagnosis needs to be undertaken as soon as possible by a qualified physician. Diagnosis will include a pelvic examination, blood tests for STIs, urinary tract infections and pregnancy, and possibly other blood tests. Other examinations may also be required, such as an ultrasound, a laparoscopy or an endometrial biopsy.

TREATMENT

The treatment of the origin of the inflammation, the bacteria or fungal infection, is usually by use of broad-spectrum antibiotics. If PID has caused adhesions then further treatment may be advised.

Other conditions that influence fertility

Diabetes

As with most species, our systems are geared to reproduction, and so many systems directly relate to this imperative. Insulin is directly related to leptin and oestrogen, and so it is not surprising that diabetes can affect fertility. Diabetes mellitus (termed as such because the urine smells sweet, like honey) is differentially diagnosed as type 1 and type 2 diabetes. Type 1 diabetes, also known as insulin-dependent diabetes, or early-onset diabetes because it develops in patients under the age of 40, is suffered by about 180 million people worldwide (WHO) and is rising at about 3 per cent per year.[23] The far more common form of diabetes, type 2, is also increasing significantly in adolescents, as the average BMI in the world population continues to soar.

The cause of diabetes is a failure of the body's system to transfer glucose from the blood into the cells. This failure occurs because either not enough insulin is being produced (it is produced by the pancreas) or hyperinsulinemia has occurred. In type 1 diabetes, the immune system is the primary culprit, destroying insulin-producing cells. In the lifestyle-determined type 2 diabetes, not enough insulin is produced or the body has become insulin resistant.

In terms of fertility, diabetes is associated with menstrual problems including oligomenorrhoea and secondary amenorrhoea, hyperandrogenism and PCOS, reduction in the reproductive period, Hashimoto's thyroiditis, anti-ovarian auto-antibodies and sexual dysfunction.

SYMPTOMS

- Feeling very thirsty
- Frequent urination, especially at night
- Exhaustion
- Weight loss and loss of muscle bulk

Treatment of diabetes requires differential diagnosis, evaluation of complications (if any) and where necessary, insulin treatment and lifestyle advice.

The thyroid

A healthy functioning thyroid is very important for fertility. The thyroid is responsible for the energy requirements of every cell and secretes thyroid hormones thyroxine (T4), triodothyronine (T3), 3,5-diiodothyronine (T2) and 3 monoiodothyronine (T1), and calcitonin. Although produced by the thyroid, the roles of T2 and T1 are not yet fully identified. Recent evidence has shown that T2 doesn't mimic the effects of T3, as previously thought, but appears to stimulate mitochondrial respiration, speed up metabolism and reduce fat storage, which is probably one of the reasons it's so popular in the body-building sport. It has been shown to stimulate the enzyme that converts T4 to T3, whilst also influencing other enzymes, ion-exchangers and the transcription of some genes.[24, 25] On the other hand, the role of T1 has remained as a precursor of T4 and T3.

Production and secretion of these hormones is prompted by the secretion of thyroid-stimulating hormone (TSH) from the pituitary. In turn, the pituitary is prompted to secrete TSH by receiving thyrotropin-releasing hormone (TRH) from the hypothalamus. The hypothalamus produces and secretes TRH in response to blood levels of T4 and T3. When levels of T4 and T3 are low, the hypothalamus secretes TRH, which instructs the pituitary to secrete TSH.

It is important that the patient is caring for her thyroid. Along with other factors, stress hormones are known to inhibit TSH and therefore impair production of T4 and T3. Although blood tests can evaluate the range of free T4 and T3, even where thyroid function does not fall within the clinically relevant range it appears to have a role in premenstrual syndrome (PMS) and also affect ovarian function.[26] Low thyroid levels will impair ovarian function and lead to impaired progesterone production. Moreover, there appears to be a relationship between low thyroid function and PCOS.

HYPOTHYROIDISM

Causes

The most common cause is iodine deficiency, which is usually a result of a diet low in iodine. Another cause often seen is autoimmune thyroiditis, where the immune system creates antibodies against the thyroid gland. What causes the immune response is unknown as yet, but it appears that a family history of hypothyroidism may indicate the potential to develop this response. Graves' disease, an enlarged thyroid gland and a history of other autoimmune diseases are also implicated. Other causes include the side effects of some medicines, a pituitary problem and congenital disease.

Symptoms

- Tiredness
- Weight gain
- Fluid retention
- Feeling cold
- Body aches
- Lustreless hair
- Constipation
- A progressive mental slowing
- Memory loss and confusion
- Depression
- Sub-fertility
- Irregular periods
- Heavy periods

HYPERTHYROIDISM

Causes

Hyperthyroidism can be differentiated into primary hyperthyroidism and secondary hyperthyroidism: primary hyperthyroidism originates within the thyroid gland; secondary hyperthyroidism originates from the pituitary.

The main cause of hyperthyroidism is the autoimmune disease, Graves' disease. Inflammation of the thyroid (thyroiditis) can be caused by autoimmune response, as in Hashimoto's thyroiditis, and also as a result of childbirth (postpartum thyroiditis), although in this latter incidence, thyroid function usually recovers quickly. In some cases, the lack of iodine in the diet can lead to toxic thyroid adenoma. On the other hand, excess iodine, or thyroid hormone consumption, can also cause hyperthyroidism, as in Graves' disease, or hamburger hyperthyroidism (ground beef, or meat from other animals, that has been contaminated by thyroid tissue in food products such as hamburgers is thought to cause hyperthyroidism, and is the most common cause of thyrotoxicosis), or overuse of thyroid hormone tablets. Side effects of some medicines (amiodarone, for instance) are also known causes.

Symptoms

- Increased heartbeat
- Weight loss or weight gain
- Increased or decreased appetite
- Irritability
- Weakness and fatigue
- Diarrhoea
- Sweating
- Tremor
- Mental illness
- Sub-fertility (amenorrhea or oligomenorrhoea)
- Loss of libido

INVESTIGATIONS OF THYROID PROBLEMS

First-line investigations for thyroid function are blood tests. The first test is usually to evaluate the levels of TSH.

Where the thyroid is compromised and working below par, the diagnosis is hypothyroidism. Production of T3 will be low, which the hypothalamus will sense and inform the pituitary that more TSH is required. Blood levels of TSH will be high. Further tests for levels of T4 and T3 will be required.

Where the thyroid is overactive and making too much T3 and T4, the hypothalamus will detect this and signal that the pituitary reduce production of TSH. Blood levels of TSH will be low. Further tests for levels of T4 and T3 will be required.

Depending on the result of the tests, other investigations may be called for, including ultrasound scans and tests to exclude autoimmune diseases.

TREATMENTS OF THYROID PROBLEMS

Treatment to help restore thyroid function includes oral administration of either T4, or T3 and T4. Depending on the result of the diagnosis, other medicines may be brought to bear, including thyrostatics (carbimazole for instance) and beta-blockers. Surgery may be required to remove the whole thyroid, or nodules that are compromising thyroid function. However, this is unusual since treatment with radioiodine can treat most forms of hyperthyroidism.

General investigations

Blood tests

SEXUALLY TRANSMITTED DISEASES

When a patient decides to try for a family, tests should include a sexually transmitted diseases (STD) blood test. Not only can many STDs interfere with attempts to become pregnant, some can cause infertility. Moreover, there is the potential that some will be passed to the foetus.

Chlamydia is a sexually transmitted disease. It has been shown to cause scarring in the fallopian tubes, is a causative factor of PID and a test should be undertaken. If the test is positive a course of antibiotics is recommended.

Other STIs to be tested for include HIV/AIDS, hepatitis, gonorrhoea, syphilis and trichomoniasis.

OESTROGEN AND PROGESTERONE

Oestrogen and progesterone blood tests help establish the hormonal balance and give an indication of how the endocrine system is working. For oestrogen, blood should be taken on day one or at the latest day two of the menstrual cycle, whereas the progesterone test should be taken seven days prior to the menstrual bleed.

OTHER HORMONE TESTS

In the event that the menstrual cycle is irregular, plasma levels of FSH and LH will be evaluated. Other hormones that may influence the regularity of the menstrual cycle are prolactin, TSH and testosterone, and it may be that these will need to be evaluated.

ANTI-MULLERIAN HORMONE TEST (OVARIAN RESERVE)

The anti-mullerian hormone (AMH) test is now common. In women, anti-mullerian hormone is secreted by granulosa cells, cells that support the development of the oocyte, folliculogenesis and ultimately, follicular atresia.

An ovarian follicle comprises a range of cells, which include granulosa cells and an oocyte. Granulosa cells are multi-function cells. It is thought they secrete factors that contribute to the maturation of the oocyte; they are stimulated by FSH, are responsible for the conversion of androgens to estradiol, and through secretion of estradiol modulate the HPO, secretion of FSH and LH, and therefore their functions influence ovulation. In the luteal phase they change both state and function, becoming granulosa lutein cells that secrete progesterone; they secrete the anti-mullerian hormone, and finally, they are implicated in follicular atresia.

Follicular atresia (from the Greek a, 'not', and 'tretos', meaning 'perforated') is the natural regulatory process whereby ovarian follicles degenerate and are subsumed back into the ovary. As the ovarian follicle increases in size, so oestrogen secretion increases. The feedback to the hypothalamus causes a reduction of FSH secretion which ultimately precipitates follicular atresia. In a fully functioning natural ovarian cycle, FSH is the key inhibitor of the process, whilst granulosa cell apoptosis, TNFα, and Fas ligand are implicated in the follicular degeneration.[27, 28]

Secretion of AMH is perceptible in primary follicles, highest in antral and pre-antral follicles, and decreases as follicle size increases, becoming practically zero by the time a follicle reaches 8mm, and is imperceptible in follicles undergoing atresia.[29]

Why is the AMH test also referred to as 'ovarian reserve'?

Follicular atresia is relentless. With each menstrual cycle rising FSH recruits a further 20 or so immature follicles of which all but the largest go through the degenerative and subsumption process associated with FSH decline. This means that the pool of remaining follicles consistently declines. The number of follicles growing at each cycle appears to be significantly dependent on the number of remaining primordial follicles.[30, 31] Since AMH is produced by follicles, and its production declines as follicles grow, blood levels of AMH are interpreted as a reflection of the size of the group of remaining primary and primordial follicles. Hence the term 'ovarian reserve'.

In general, an AMH test provides a guide for the number of follicles that will result from an IVF cycle. A higher AMH result is interpreted as potentially better for a patient simply in terms of response to ovarian hyperstimulation, although there are a few confounding factors. For instance, a woman with polycystic ovaries will have many smaller follicles and therefore have a higher AMH reading.

An AMH test does not identify the quality of the egg.

Genetic tests

Genetic tests can be advised for a variety of reasons. These include the presence of current or suspected hereditary diseases, such as thalassaemia and sickle cell, or to try to identify the cause of failed IVF cycles or recurrent miscarriage. A recent study undertaken at the Peninsula Medical School showed that, in future, it may be possible to genetically identify the reproductive span of a woman through a blood test.[32]

Another area where considerable interest is shown is the new technology of PGD. This technology is brought to bear when there is a hereditary disease, or when a couple have had a child with a serious genetic condition, or when there have been multiple pregnancy losses. It has also been used to identify the sex of the child.

The HFEA lists over one hundred conditions where PGD can be used, although it is down to the clinic to judge whether the test should be employed or not. In the UK, to undertake such a test the clinic must have a licence and adhere to the code of practice provided by the HFEA. Clinics with such a licence are permitted to test for any condition, or any group of conditions that are published on the HFEA list of PGD conditions. The exception to this rule is human leukocyte antigens (HLA) tissue typing which can only be approved by the HFEA, and only on a case-by-case basis.

HLA tissue typing, more commonly referred to as pre-implantation tissue typing (PTT) and also known through the media as 'saviour siblings', is used when there is a serious life-threatening genetic disorder, for example Diamond Blackfan anaemia (DBA) or beta thalassemia (BTM). Patients suffering from DBA or BTM require regular and frequent blood transfusions, iron chelation and, in some cases, bone marrow transplantation.

The parents of a child born with such a condition may apply to the HFEA to conceive another child, a 'saviour' child. A 'saviour' child is conceived to provide an organ or a cell transplant for his/her sibling. IVF is the only way to do this. After conception, the PGD is carried out to ensure (a) that the siblings are genetically compatible and (b) that the genetic disease is excluded.

Imaging tests

A hysterosalpingogram is a type of x-ray taken of the womb and fallopian tubes. A dye is injected that delineates the outline of the womb and any blockage of the fallopian tubes.

HyCoSy is a procedure that involves the injection of fluid into the womb. The ultrasound detects whether the fluid spills out of the fallopian tubes, thereby identifying any blockages. However, even with this technique, blockages can be difficult to identify.

A laparoscopy is a more invasive procedure and is advised if there is a history of a previous problem, such as if the patient has previously suffered a pelvic inflammatory disease. The laparoscope is inserted through a small incision in the lower abdomen to observe the womb, ovaries and fallopian tubes. A dye is often injected into the fallopian tubes through the cervix to identify the presence of any blockages.

6

Lifestyle

The Stress Epidemic and Stress Hormones

Any discussion about lifestyle and fertility must begin with stress. Studies show that stress is caused by sub-fertility and in some studies has been shown to be caused by the treatment of sub-fertility. However, research evaluating the effect of stress on fertility and IVF outcomes is still inconclusive. The difference in results may be due to different types of stress activation leading to different stress pathways, different types of stress per se and the individual response, that is, different individual lifestyles and different capabilities to resist stress and the effect of stress (resilience). Whatever the ultimate cause, many studies show elevation in stress hormones, and dysregulation of the fertility axis as a result of individual response to stress and fertility. The net result is that commentators are now suggesting that fertility treatment should begin by treating stress.

There is an ancient Chinese saying: 'May you live in interesting times.' In the West this saying is often misunderstood, and thought to be a blessing. In fact, traditional thought from long ago understood that interesting times can impair health and life expectancy. Interesting times can be stressful.

National stress

It's not quite the elephant in the room that no one is mentioning but, actually, is it? How much stress are people facing now? In the UK, a survey from 2005 showed that 79 per cent of UK citizens felt they were stressed. Worryingly, more than a third of men and more than a quarter of women stated they rely on alcohol to help manage stress.[1] In 2011, a popular newspaper emphasised the dangers of stress with an article stating that stress in the UK is considered equivalent to the Black Death.[2] The word 'stress', when used by the Health and Safety Executive (HSE), means 'stress, depression or anxiety'. The data sources used are the Labour Force Survey created by the Office of National Statistics, and the THOR GP scheme. The HSE publication, Stress and Psychological Disorders in Great Britain 2013, reported on information derived from 2011 to 2012, which showed that from 2011 to 2012 roughly 40 per cent of workplace illness was workplace stress (about 428,000 people suffered from stress, depression or anxiety of a total of 1,073,000 of work related illness).[3] When the statistics are sorted by gender, the HSE report a total of 175,000 men and 253,000 women suffering from work-related stress between 2011 and 2012.[4]

In 2008, just over 22 per cent of the Canadian population reported being highly stressed. In 2011 this figure had increased to nearly 24 per cent. One in five Canadians are suffering from stress-related mental health problems, and depression in Canada is on its way to becoming the leading disability.[5]

In the US, from 2007 to 2010 stress increased so much that, in terms of stress levels and the number of US citizens dealing with it, the American Psychological Association warned of a public health crisis.[6] The Stress in America survey 2012 found that the overall stress levels were down in comparison to the preceding year, but that 35 per cent of respondents felt their stress had increased and 20 per cent reported extreme stress. In America 23 per cent of women are living with extreme stress, compared to 16 per cent of men. Since the chances of premature death are increased by 16 per cent for people who experience low-level anxiety and stress, and the chances are significantly increased where the experience of stress and anxiety is higher, it is no wonder the American Psychological Association are worried.[7]

We know that stress is bad for us. Sudden death following a serious traumatic event or acute stress has been observed for a long time. Coronary heart disease (CHD), also known as coronary artery disease or atherosclerotic heart disease, is much more common in people living with chronic stress. Men who regularly experience even moderate stress events over a number of years are in significant danger; the early mortality rate for this group is 50 per cent higher than in men experiencing low stress events.[8] Several years ago, the association between chronic stress and heart disease was identified as a risk factor for police officers in New York and other cities. Coronary heart disease is the most common cause of death in the world,[9] and is the number one cause of death of women in the US.

Recent evidence shows that stress causes an increase in stress hormones, which in turn results in increased coronary artery calcification (CAC). CAC is a marker for coronary heart disease. Although medical opinion is still to come to a firm conclusion about the relationship between stress and CHD, and some of the reasons are due to the diversity of potential etiologies, individual resilience and response to stressors, as research methodology and investigative techniques become more sophisticated, it's probable that a definitive link will soon be found.

Excluding its impact on fertility, stress has been linked to over one hundred other medical conditions, either as a primary cause or as an associative factor. These include depression, anxiety attacks, alcoholism, substance abuse, chronic fatigue syndrome, insulin resistance, hypothyroidism, psoriasis, fibromyalgia, arrhythmia, Alzheimer's diease, Parkinson's disease, Cushing's disease, type 2 diabetes[10] and many more.

Origins of stress

We have come a long way since the term 'stress' was first created. It was Hans Seyle from whom this term originated. As a result of his experiments, Seyle initially developed a theory of stress, which he named as the 'General Adaptation Syndrome' and which he later called the Stress Response. He initially defined stress as 'the non-specific neuroendocrine response of the body to any demand for change' from which definition he later dropped 'neuroendocrine, and went on to identify some of the biochemicals involved in the stress response, including adrenaline (epinephrine), noradrenaline (norepinephrine) and cortisol (hydrocortisone or cortisone).[11]

Stress is differentiated into categories such as acute stress, where the fight/flight response is initiated to manage an acute stressor; chronic stress, where continual low levels of stress are aroused to manage one or many continuously concurrent low-level stressors; and post-traumatic stress, where a prior event causes a consistent acute stress state. I believe a fourth category should be added to this, called burnout.

The etiologies of stress are varied and include work, relationships, social situation, finances, health problems and a lack of control over one's life. Recently, commentators have put forward four key categories as a further concept of the causation of stress. These are: novel, unpredictable and uncontrollable situations, or threats to the individual from their society (e.g. social rejection).[12] If we consider what a couple faces when starting sub-fertility treatment, it's quite easy to see that all four of these categories apply to IVF.

Stress as a motivator

Not all stress is bad. In fact, a normal and reasonable level of stress hormones is required; cortisol secretion is elevated early in the morning for a reason, and for working life, a reasonable amount of motivation/arousal is also necessary if we are going to achieve anything during our day. This latter point originates from Yerkes and Dodson.

Yerkes Dodson law (1908) states that performance is correlated with arousal, but that increases or decreases in arousal will eventually be deleterious to performance. Since its origination, the knowledge base has increased and arousal can be thought of as both physiological and emotional arousal. In this context, arousal is often used synonymously with stress, but the discrimination is in the detail; early in the performance process, and until the peak, arousal relates to a group of physical changes including increased heart rate indicating elevated hormonal state similar to a stress response. In addition, as we would expect, both physiological and cognitive capabilities, such as memory, intention, expectation and motivation, are also increased.[13] However, both acute and chronic stress eventuate in a reduction in these latter capabilities.

The relationship between performance and arousal is easiest to appreciate graphically; on a graph the x axis identifies performance and the y axis identifies arousal. The Yerkes Dodson law states that where arousal outstrips performance, performance will decline, so the graph is bell shaped.

Operating at peak performance is not a novel concept; Maslow investigated it and following Maslow, the work of Mihaly

Csikszentmihalyi during 1970s led to the development of flow psychology. At some stage during a working event performance will peak; creative, physical, emotional and/or mental capacities will cohere in a unity, working in a concerted flow to fulfil potential, peak performance. An illustration Csikszentmihalyi uses is skiing; to operate at peak performance, the skier must be entirely focused on the run – there is no room for extraneous concerns. Importantly, Csikszentmihalyi states that these moments are not limited to physical exercise, or to work, but extend over the range of social interaction. It is, in fact, a way of life. The amount of time a person can stay at peak performance depends on the individual and, the longer it is, the longer the performance plateau will be. Ultimately though, the capacity to perform will begin to decrease.

In the work-related environment, arousal is often identified as motivation: as motivation increases, so performance increases until the individual reaches peak performance. If motivation continues to increase, the individual takes on more tasks than can be reasonably handled, so performance begins to decline until eventually the number of tasks become overwhelming.

Work-related stress

Work is identified as a major cause of stress. This key stress domain draws in categories such as finances, social concerns and environmental factors. Lack of control over one's working life is commonly cited. Stress caused by work is the main cause of workplace sickness. Data from the Whitehall II study, which included more than 10,000 male and female participants, concluded that work-related stress may be a key factor in coronary heart disease and a dysregulation of the HPA.[14, 15] In fact, so much data has been unearthed about the relationship between health and work, including psychiatric disorders, depressive disorders and cortisol awakening response, that the Whitehall II study is worth taking a good long look at.[16]

Working, stress and women's health

The effects of stress differ between individuals and between genders; men are more likely to initiate the fight/flight reflex, whereas women are more likely to take care of themselves either directly or by increasing social interaction. In many cases it appears that women are better at establishing self-care and developing coping strategies to illness than men;[17] where personal nurture is inhibited or insufficient, extending social networks and nurturing others can also be a beneficial way to manage stress, a model referred to as 'tend and befriend'.[18] Obviously one cares for one's friends. Moreover, the sense of isolation (a common experience of illness in the West, and a stress factor) is reduced by extending one's social connections.

The gender difference may be due to a combination of both nature and nurture; the hormone oxytocin is much more prevalent in female physiology than in male physiology, and from a sociological view, men are more likely to communicate competitively, whereas women are more likely communicate supportively. A large study of 1100 adults found that compared to men, women were more vulnerable to depression, and more likely to experience chronic strain and less mastery over their lives. Women were also more likely to ruminate. The authors found that ruminating and lack of mastery of life increases vulnerability to depressive symptoms, as does ruminating and chronic strain, and simultaneous experience of chronic strain, lack of mastery and ruminating also exacerbates vulnerability to depressive symptoms.[19, 20]

In 2009, in Canada, over 25 per cent of women reported their life stress was 'quite a bit' or 'extreme'.[21] Women who report high job stress have a 40 per cent higher risk of cardiovascular disease than their lower-stress peers. The fear of job loss is associated in women with risk factors for high blood pressure, increased cholesterol and excess body weight. Women who don't go out to work seem to be better off in terms of stress compared to women who do and it appears that work-related stress may affect IVF outcome.[22, 23]

Neurohormonal factors

At the biochemical level, in response to a homeostatic threat, the sympathetic nervous system causes the secretion of a range of neurohormones including adrenaline, noradrenaline and cortisol.

Earlier, we discussed the relationship between the hypothalamus, the pituitary and the ovaries – the HPO axis – and we saw how closely related they are, and how the messaging system caused adaption in each organ. The HPA axis is similar, although instead of the ovaries, the adrenal glands are the third member of the triangle.

Cortisol/hydrocortisone: $C_{21}H_{30}O_5$

Cortisol is quite possibly the most potent of steroids. Also known as hydrocortisone, or simply cortisone, it is a steroid hormone that is produced and secreted by the adrenal glands – in the outer layer of the adrenal glands, the adrenal cortex.

Both acute and chronic low-level cortisol secretion appear able to inhibit LH and FSH secretion, and this inhibition may be at either the pituitary or the hypothalamic level via suppression of GnRH. However, inhibition and the level of inhibition may once again depend on individual resilience to stress.

Cortisol follows a frequency pattern that is diurnal. Secretion starts to decrease in the evening and is lowest in the small hours, between 12am and 4am, and peaks between 7am and 8am. It is a glucocorticoid, which is a group of steroids that play a role in the metabolism of glucose. Glucocorticoids perform several functions, one of which is modulation of the immune system to reduce inflammation.

In response to stress, hydrocortisone is secreted to increase blood sugar, reduce inflammation by suppressing the immune system and enhance metabolic rate. The secretion is triggered at the hypothalamic level and secreted by the hypothalamus; corticotropin-releasing hormone (CRH) triggers the pituitary secretion of adrenocorticotropic hormone (ACTH), which is carried to the adrenals and subsequently triggers cortisol secretion.

The action of cortisol on the receptor for IL-2 inhibits production of B-cell antibody mediated inflammation, hence its use in inflammatory conditions such as allergies and eczema. B-cells are a member of the lymphocyte family of white blood cells, which bind to an antibody against an antigen. However, in association with IL-10 a branch of B-cells (Bregs) regulates the immune system and suppresses inflammation.[24] In so doing, cortisol diverts energy from the immune system, a low priority system in the fight/flight response. It also supports adrenaline (and noradrenaline) in the catabolisation of glycogen to glucose. In this way more glucose is available for the brain and new energy is transferred from storage (adipose tissue).

Since it is involved in glucose production and glucose levels in the blood, it is right to think that cortisol influences insulin. In the periphery, cortisol encourages insulin resistance, and at the same time encourages the creation of glucose from non-carbohydrates in the liver, a process often relied upon in body-building circles and termed glucoseneogenesis.

In general, chronically elevated cortisol is also associated with decreases in muscle growth, sex drive, bone density, cardiovascular health and healthy sleep. In people aged 65 and over, elevated cortisol levels increase the chances of death from a cardiovascular event by a factor of five.[25] The catabolisation of protein is most evident in the depletion of collagen, the main protein in connective tissue, and collagen depreciation from skin is significantly greater than from other tissue.[26]

Elevated cortisol is a known risk factor for fertility at the neuroendocrine level. When cortisol becomes elevated, fertility declines and in some cases the reproductive system shuts down altogether. This effect may occur through many pathways: at the hypothalamic level and interfering with the HPO; by elevation of prolactin, thereby dysregulating ovulation; by modulating the immune system and dysregulating implantation; and by directly affecting the uterus and fallopian tubes though neuronal excitation.

Progesterone is an indirect precursor of cortisol. Where cortisol levels are increased so progesterone may be influenced: this may play a role in corpus luteal development, endometrial receptivity and luteal phase defect. Elevated cortisol is also implicated in unruptured follicle syndrome (UFS).

Chronic stress appears to reduce IVF outcome, and chronically elevated cortisol is known to either cause or be implicated in conditions that affect fertility.[27, 28] These include endocrine disorders (such as Cushing's syndrome), endometriosis, and the most common cause of sub-fertility, PCOS. Some studies have shown that both stress and mood are strongly implicated in PCOS, and there is a strong associative connection between chronically elevated cortisol and insulin resistance.

The relationship between cortisol and insulin means we must look at leptin. As we know, leptin is directly required for reproduction.

Leptin and cortisol share a circadian rhythm pattern, although it is an inverse relationship: leptin levels are higher at night when cortisol levels are low, and during the day leptin levels are low when cortisol levels are high. Leptin may be the yin to cortisol's yang, although cortisol's circadian rhythm is based on light and dark, whereas leptin's is based on food and not-food.

The association of leptin with hypothalamic CRH expression, and in the adrenals with ACTH means that it shares a pathway with cortisol, and through that pathway an indirect relationship with the catecholamines.

A dysfunctional relationship between leptin and cortisol was identified in the last century and is still thought to be a prevailing cause of metabolic syndrome (also known as syndrome X, and in Australia, as CHAOS), thought to affect 25 per cent of US citizens. Diagnostic symptoms of this syndrome include insulin resistance, PCOS, type 2 diabetes, high blood pressure and central obesity (significant weight gain in the centre, e.g. pot belly/beer belly).

Both leptin and insulin are fundamentally involved in the development of obesity and it now appears that cortisol has a significant role in this epidemic. Cortisol modulates leptin and insulin, leptin is involved in cortisol secretion and also modulates insulin, and elevated cortisol appears to elevate leptin secretion.[29] Chronically elevated leptin (and leptin resistance) will eventually lead to insulin resistance. The energy has to go somewhere, and when cells become insensitive to insulin, that port is no longer available, so the energy is transferred to storage as fat. This triangle between cortisol, leptin and insulin is probably one of the reasons for the failure of fad diets.

In addition to a range of medical conditions associated with PCOS, such as depression, high blood pressure, and hyperglycaemia and obesity, both metabolic syndrome and insulin resistance are highly correlated with PCOS and it is thought that insulin resistance could be a primary cause of this syndrome. In fact, the correlation appears to be so close that many think PCOS and insulin resistance should be considered concurrently.[30]

Although normal cortisol secretion may have a positive effect on oocyte maturation and early pregnancy, evidence shows that elevated cortisol may be responsible for very early pregnancy loss, that is, pregnancy loss within the first three weeks.[31] Whether this is in response to a chronic situation or an acute one is yet to be determined.

Adrenaline/epinephrine: $C_9H_{13}NO_3$

Adrenaline is both a hormone and a neurotransmitter. It is secreted by the adrenal glands, specifically the medulla of the adrenal gland, and some neurons in the central nervous system (CNS). Adrenaline secretion becomes elevated in response to potential threats to homeostasis. The production process is initially oxidation of tyrosine to L-DOPA (the precursor of dopamine and noradrenaline/norepinephrine) to produce noradrenaline. Noradrenaline undergoes a further (catalytic) reaction to produce adrenaline.

Adrenaline is a thoroughly important hormone for many of our physiological processes. In response to a threat and in concert with cortisol, adrenaline promotes glycogenolysis, that is, the creation of glucose from glycogen. It inhibits insulin secretion so that cells in the liver, muscles and adipose tissue are prevented from absorbing glucose from blood. More energy is freely available to help the body and mind deal with the perceived threat.

Elevated epinephrine influences blood flow: it is a vasodilator, dilating smooth muscle tissues lining the airways, and at the same time causes contraction of smooth muscle tissue that lines blood vessels between arteries and capillaries, arterioles. These actions reduce blood flow to the exterior, whilst preserving blood flow in the core. A key factor in the fight/flight response is to protect the core.

Like monocytes/macrophages which 'learn' and 'store' the physiological data from bacteria, viruses and other organisms harmful to our system, the monoamine adrenaline enhances memory of stressful circumstances. The memory of such events can find expression autonomically; in increased heartbeat and palpitations, and through both cognitive memory and emotional memory.

Noradrenaline/norepinephrine: $C_8H_{11}NO_3$

Noradrenaline/norepinephrine is a hormone and a neurotransmitter. It is part of the monoamine/catecholamine system and is derived from its precursor L DOPA, also the precursor to dopamine, another monoamine and catecholamine. It becomes elevated in response to stress and low blood pressure (which also threatens homeostasis) from the sympathetic nervous system and from the adrenal glands, specifically, the adrenal medulla.

It is an excellent hormone for the fight/flight response. It increases heart rate, contractions and thereby blood flow, and increases blood pressure by increasing the tension in vascular smooth muscle tissue. Like epinephrine, it increases the availability of glucose supply from storage, and blood flow to skeletal muscle, once again protecting the core.

Norepinephrine also affects our emotional and cognitive abilities. The noradrenergic system projects from areas in the brain related to reward (e.g. sex and feeding behaviours) into areas related to violence and the control of violence. The system also projects from another area in the brain, the locus coeruleus, which is related to cognitive functions. Attention deficit hyperactivity disorder (ADHD) medications, such as the selective noradrenaline reuptake inhibitor (SNRI), atomoxetine (brand name Straterra), and methylphenidate (brand name Ritalin), effectively increase levels of norepinephrine, although it is still not exactly understood how methyphenidate works and it is thought that serotonin may be implicated.[32]

The medical condition depression can be caused by stress and iatrogenically by the reductive action of some drugs on monoamines in the brain.[33] A deficiency of noradrenaline is strongly associated with depression, as is serotonin, and SSRIs (like Prozac) inhibit the reuptake of both serotonin and noradrenaline to sustain their presence in the body.

Excitement, excitement hormones and reactive species

Dopamine: $C_8H_{11}NO_2$

The precursor of dopamine is L-DOPA, so it shares the same root with the catecholamines discussed earlier in this chapter. Like the others, it is a monoamine, a neurotransmitter and a hormone found throughout the body, produced in the brain and locally. It is not an excitatory molecule; rather, it appears to reduce nerve signal transmission. Dopamine is almost entirely diurnal in its secretory pattern.

The secretion of noradrenalin in the periphery is regulated by dopamine, by binding to receptors in the arterial walls, which inhibits noradrenalin release and promotes vasodilatation. In this way dopamine works in concert with noradrenaline to increase blood flow. Dopamine also inhibits the secretion of the hormone prolactin, secretion of which is known to be increased by stress and, along with other biochemicals, and adrenaline.[34]

Dopamine is associated with the immune system through modulation of lymphocyte activation, and with blood sugar by modulating insulin secretion, and with the kidneys by increasing kidney function, particularly excretion of sodium, and by improving blood flow. In this latter attribute, it could be considered to have anti-hypertensive properties.

Secretion of dopamine is increased when a reward is received or an achievement is reached; a person with high secretion of dopamine will derive more pleasure from achievement and therefore be more motivated to repeat the experience. It is also associated with attention span. Too little can cause memory loss and is associated with schizophrenia and adult ADHD. Dopamine is associated with other mental, emotional and physiological effects including nausea, lactation, motivation and arousal, and sexual gratification.

Dopamine also modulates reactive oxygen species (ROS); when dopamine excess peaks, ROS and apoptosis (meaning pre-programmed cell death/suicide)* are elevated, whereas it has been found that when dopamine levels are low, concomitantly lower levels of intracellular ROS and ROS-derived apoptosis are shown.[35]

MEDICAL CONDITIONS ASSOCIATED WITH DOPAMINE

Dopamine is involved in many medical conditions, including Parkinson's disease, schizophrenia, ADHD and restless legs syndrome. In women, inappropriate dopamine regulation at the hypothalamic level may be involved in the dysregulation of

* The term apoptosis is derived from the combination of two Greek words: apo, translated as 'separation',[36] and ptosis, translated as 'falling off'.[37] The transliterated sense of the combination of the two words is 'the falling off of leaves' or 'pieces of leaves'.[38] This sense is also applied in biology where the death/suicide of the cell 'liberates small bodies'.[39]

gonadotropins, indicating that dopamine may be pathogenically implicated in PCOS.

Circadian rhythm, sleep and vulnerability to substance abuse appear significantly connected, and dopamine and elevated cortisol are probably key in this relationship. Disrupted sleep patterns are both a cause of stress, by circadian rhythm disruption causing a similar disruption in circadian-regulated secretion of dopamine and cortisol, and caused by stress by the same dynamic.

Goal setting is a good example of the relationship between motivation and dopamine. When we achieve something, dopamine is secreted, donating a sense of pleasure at the achievement. When we set a goal, emotionally, psychologically and neurologically we are creating an event within ourselves. We can see the goal, which means that even if externally we haven't achieved the goal, internally we have. So, our motivation is empowered by the need to realise (make real) the goal. An example of this is setting the internal clock; at night, just before going to sleep, many people set their internal clock to wake at a certain time. Providing no disrupting influences have been consumed (i.e. alcohol or a sleeping pill) many people achieve this goal and report a sensation of satisfaction on waking.

DOPAMINIC WAVE

Dopamine secretion fluctuates in frequency and amplitude according to internal and external influences. Some short time after increases in dopamine secretion peak, at the crest, so there is a natural return down the other side of the wave. Think of when you last achieved something significant. Once the initial sense of satisfaction has subsided we return back down from the crest to our normal emotional world. What would happen to us if our lifestyle, our living circumstances, perpetuated over a long period of time a consistently rapid, frequent return to the crest? Could we ever return to a normal emotional world?

Dopamine is increased when particular drugs are taken, like cocaine and methamphetamines. An evocative description I have recently read of the effect of dopamine depletion is that suffered by people addicted to meth. Meth initially increases dopamine whilst preventing reuptake. So the taker experiences an extenuated crest of euphoria. The trough is a reflection of the crest and so a deep low, a depression, is experienced as the effects of the drug wear off. This experience enhances the addictive nature of the drug and repeated use will eventuate in the withering of dopamine receptors and reuptake sites, which are eventually extirpated. For the meth addict, most sense of the world other than monochrome is eventually extinguished.

Serotonin (5-hydroxytryptophan/5-HT): $C_{10}H_{12}N_{20}$

Serotonin (5-HT) is another monoamine neurotransmitter and hormone, but with serotinergic neurons derived mostly from the area in the brain relating to attention, motivation and emotion, the raphe nucleus. Serotonin is mostly found in the gastrointestinal tract. It is a subtle but pervasive transmitter and its actions are dependent on its receptors, of which there are several. From a biological perspective, serotonin not only influences the rate of intercellular communication but also the secretion of a range of neurotransmitters. On an emotional/mind level, it is involved in the expression of a range of emotions including anxiety, appetite, sexual behaviour, cognitive abilities, memory and mood.

Depression is one of the fastest growing disabilities and the range of the world's population suffering from depression has increased significantly. In 1990 major depressive disorder was the fourth leading cause of global disability, by 2000 it was the leading cause of non-fatal burden, and 2010 it was ranked second largest contributor to the burden of disease in the global burden of disease study.[40, 41] Previously, depression was a condition mostly suffered by the elderly; the average age of sufferers is now 30 and it is a common disability in teenagers.

Serotonin appears to share the responsibility for this condition with noradrenaline and dopamine. Although the majority of treatment is with SSRIs, which target serotonin, they can weakly influence noradrenaline and dopamine. More recent pharmacological development has produced SNRIs, which are used to treat a range of conditions other than depression including ADHD, fibromyalgia and climacteric symptoms suffered during menopause. The side effects of these drugs include loss of appetite, weight loss, sleep problems, sexual dysfunction and loss of libido, and potentially high blood pressure.

The role of calcium

In the fight/flight response, an increased heart rate is common. Intracellular calcium is primarily responsible for contractility and increased intracellular calcium increases the contraction of heart muscle, and therefore heart rate. Calcium is an absolute cellular necessity, and so there is a mechanism that permits calcium entrance to cells.

Both adrenaline and noradrenaline increase intracellular calcium through their activation of the enzyme adenyl cyclase, which permits phosphorylation and opening of voltage-dependent calcium channels (VDCCs), ion channels membranes of cells that are capable of being excited. The opening of these channels is dependent on cellular depolarisation.

The concentration of calcium outside the cell is significantly greater than within the cell (and here we're talking of an order of magnitude several thousand times greater) so, when a VDCC is activated, calcium rushes into the cell. Amongst other outcomes, the influx causes muscle contraction. This is great when a response is needed, but what happens when the ingressive rush of calcium becomes excessive?

Excitotoxicity

Balance is a by-word in many cultures. Excitatory neurotransmitters, like glutamate or aspartate, are very important in the humdrum routine maintenance of cellular life. But when there's too much excitement, or too much of an excitatory neurotransmitter, we are looking at triggering a problem that, unless corrected, will become dangerous.

Glutamate is probably the most potent endogenous excitatory neurotransmitter. It's implicated in memory and long-term potentiation, that is, it sustains the signal and indicates signal volume between two neurons (hence glutamate is also implicated in learning); it is deeply involved in cellular metabolism, is responsible for dealing with cellular waste (getting rid of excess nitrogen) and is the precursor to the excitatory inhibitor, GABA (y-aminobutyric acid). In the synaptic cleft, glutamate secretion increases and decreases very rapidly (think milliseconds). If this process is disturbed or disrupted, and glutamate cannot be decreased or is elevated, the neuron dies; it kills itself, a process called apoptosis. Elevation of glutamate levels can occur through several mechanisms: through choice (i.e. dietary intake) or external accidents, or endogenous accidents, such as a cerebrovascular accident (stroke).

Excitatory biochemicals cause VDCCs to open. When the activation of VDCCs extends beyond normal, an excessive amount of calcium enters the cell. This is going to cause damage. Excess intercellular calcium causes enzymatic activation, which in addition to neuronal apoptosis, corrupts cellular structures, cellular mechanisms, and even structural changes to DNA. Excitotoxicity is directly implicated in a number of medical conditions such as multiple sclerosis, Alzheimer's disease, Parkinson's disease, chronic fatigue syndrome, stroke, fibromyalgia, alcoholism and alcohol withdrawal.

Many substances in the food chain can be termed excitotoxins, that is, substances that cause excitotoxicity. These include glutamate, monosodium glutamate and aspartame. More details on this are contained in the dietary section in Chapter 8.

Excess intercellular calcium can also open mitochondria (from the Greek *mito*, meaning 'thread', and *chondrion*, meaning 'granule'), or permeability membranes. Mitochondria will absorb too much calcium, causing them to expand and secrete ROS, which are free radicals. Free radicals require antioxidants to regulate them.

Reactive oxygen species

Reactive oxygen species (ROS) are molecules that contain oxygen and are a normal by-product of cellular metabolism. There are three forms of this species: superoxide dismutase (O_2), hydrogen peroxide (H_2O_2) and hydroxyl (OH). ROS are involved in the physiology and pathology of female and male fertility.

ROS are regulated by antioxidants, among other systems. Excess intracellular calcium will see excess ROS secreted. The advent of excess secretion of ROS is a threat to homeostasis, so stress, derived from ROS, has occurred. Oxidative stress is diagnosed when ROS levels are greater than the total antioxidant capacity (TAC) or specific ROS are greater than their corresponding antioxidant regulators. ROS cause damage to cellular signalling, proteins, lipids,

DNA, RNA and nerves. Oxidative stress is part of the process of aging. We are aged faster by stress.

Whilst aging affects the entire system, tissues that are subject to oxidative stress age faster than other tissues, thus exacerbating the aging process. For example, memory declines with age, but excess ROS secretion can lead to a more rapid decrease in memory and cognitive dysfunction. Alzheimer's is also accompanied by excess ROS secretion. Given that the brain requires so much oxygen to do its work, and has relatively little antioxidant defence, it is unsurprising that it can be so sensitive to oxidative stress.

High levels of ROS are implicated in many disease processes. Apart from the endogenous factors leading to elevated expression of ROS, exogenous factors can also elevate them. An example of this is diet; overeating for instance, or chronic consumption of energy-dense foods (foods high in sugar and fat) can elevate ROS and eventually cause insulin resistance. Thus, in female reproduction ROS can cause dysregulation of ovarian function, follicular maturation and corpus luteum development, and can lead to poor response in natural and assisted conception rates. Oxidative stress is also implicated in the decline of fertility that is associated with age.

Reactive nitrogen species, the other species

The other reactive species is the reactive nitrogen species (RNS). They are implicated in a range of medical conditions, including atherosclerosis, the leading cause of heart attacks. The two primary species are nitric oxide (NO) and nitric dioxide (NO_2). Nitric oxide is not the same as nitrous oxide, euphemistically called 'laughing gas', which is also now known to be the main ozone-depleting substance. The production of NO by its synthases was discussed earlier.

NO is a potent vasodilator and is involved in many aspects of female reproduction, including ovulation, endometrial vascularity and endometrial receptivity in the peri-implantation stage, implantation and pregnancy. In the presence of L-arginine, the enzymes of NO (endothelial nitric oxide synthase [eNOS], neuronal NO synthase [nNOS] and inducible NO synthase [iNOS]) produce NO by catalysis. As a free radical, NO significantly damages cells and tissues, proteins and lipids, and can be toxic. It is implicated in the pathogenesis of endometriosis, steroidogenesis and follicular development. In this latter category, NO derived from follicles has been associated with poor embryo quality and poor embryo cleavage.

Both ROS and RNS are involved in intracellular signalling. Follicular rupture relies on a range of factors that include cross talk between cytokines and ROS and RNS. Cross talk between mother and embryo is also necessary for implantation and ROS are implicated in failed implantation and placentation. In addition, excess ROS appear to increase embryo fragmentation and reduce early embryo survival rates. Some research has also found that excess ROS expression may cause the alteration of gene expression leading to impairment of early embryo development.[42, 43, 44, 45]

Increasingly, results from research show that oxidative stress can cause anxiety, although the direct link has yet to be elucidated. This is unsurprising really, since oxidative stress is a threat to homeostasis and so, at some level at the very least, the threat must be acknowledged and distress will be experienced. The correlation between oxidative stress and emotional stress and anxiety disorders suggests that it might lead to HPA dysfunction, thereby exacerbating stress and anxiety.

7

Take Back Control Part 1

Habits and Coping Mechanisms

Habits are key in our life. As regards this book, habits are also key to reduce stress and improve reproductive capacity.

Anxiety is probably the most prevalent disorder in the US. It is estimated that nearly 30 per cent of the US population suffers from anxiety disorders.[1]

Stress due to work is derived from a variety of factors. In addition to the neuroendocrine factors, lack of exercise, lack of control, unhealthy dietary habits (as in skipping meals, or relying on energy-dense food), insomnia and repeated stressful circumstances contribute to the inability to reproduce.

Stress is addictive. Increases in stress are associated with addiction, and stress itself can be addictive – we talk about adrenaline junkies, stress addicts, addictive behaviour patterns. The stress response is thought to provide the same rush as nicotine.

Lack of control is also one of the main complaints of patients undergoing IVF.

Coping mechanisms

Chronic stress is also associated with obesity. That levels of obesity in the US have reached epidemic proportions[2] might well correlate with the levels of stress that US citizens are currently suffering. Elevated cortisol appears to increase consumption of readily available energy-dense foods – sweet and high in fat – and has been shown to correlate with an increase in leptin and a reduction in insulin sensitivity.[3] Interestingly, a high WHR in women is also linked to unhealthy stress-induced cortisol secretion.[4]

Exercise

Exercise is a good way to reduce stress. Exercise causes endorphin secretion. Endorphins are endogenous (from the Greek *endo* meaning 'within' and *genis* meaning 'generating') opioids that make us feel good. The word itself is a combination of 'endogenous' and 'morphine', identifying its analgesic properties. When we exert ourselves, endorphins are secreted from the pituitary into the blood stream, into the spinal cord and brain to bind with their receptors. However, not much enters the brain, due to the blood–brain barrier.

Exercise has an effect on mood; it can uplift a person and have a positive effect on personality and self-esteem. It's reported that exercise is beneficial for depression, anxiety and stress. The results of research studies suggest that in the treatment of major depression, fast walking for 30 minutes three times a week over four months was at least as good as taking SSRIs only, or as good as taking SSRIs and exercising over the same time period. After the study ended, participants were followed up for a further six months; relapse in those that continued to exercise was 8 per cent, compared to either medicated or medicated and exercise groups,[5] in which relapse was observed in over 30 per cent. Mild or moderate major depressive disorder (MDD) can be alleviated by aerobic exercise, in a dose-dependent manner – the dose being in line with public health recommendations.[6]

Both chronic and acute anxiety symptoms are relieved by exercise, although it appears that aerobic exercise seems to be the key, and at least 21 minutes of aerobic activity is required per day.[7]

Almost any exercise will do, however – walking, swimming, yoga, tai chi. It doesn't have to be strenuous, although strenuous activity will burn muscular energy stores (glycogen). In the past, concerns were voiced that too much exercise may dysregulate reproductive function in women. Many female athletes become anovulatory during their intense training regimes and it has been thought that it was the stress of exercise that caused this. This could be due to the effects of exercise on cortisol and the subsequent effects of elevated cortisol on LH pulsatility. Recently, commentators have suggested that it has much more to do with diet, low energy reserves, and the syndrome known as the Female Athlete Triad.[8] For more information on this, the international coalition on the

Female Athlete Triad provides a wide range of position stands from athletic bodies and the International Olympic Committee Medical Commission, with guidance and advice.[9]

Diet

DIETARY HABITS

Eating breakfast has been found to have a positive influence on cardiovascular health, and has subsequently been found to improve the regulation of blood sugar and cortisol.[10]

Carbohydrates eaten during exercise modulate many endocrinological factors and glucocorticoids to inhibit consumption of stores of glycogen. High protein diets (like the Atkins diet) are not a good idea when exercising.

DIET AND DIETARY SUPPLEMENTS

In traditional thought, energy is derived from the air we breathe and the food we eat and this concept corresponds very well with modern thought.

In many cases, diet is habitual. The daily choice of foods to consume often relies on learnt behaviour that in many cases is unexamined. The process of diet implies not simply which foods are chosen, but also the way they are eaten and when. In many cases, this process is unconscious, a habit formed in the earliest of days.

Habits are made, grown, evolved; even at a genetic or at an epigenetic level, habits are formed. From the earliest of days, children learn from their environment, soak in information, acquire behavioural patterns initially from parental example, then peers, and consistently modify them in response to the evolution of their *shen*. (*Shen* is a traditional Chinese term that is translated as 'Spirit' and/or 'Mind'. In traditional terms, *shen* is made by the essence someone is born with [pre-birth energy] and the energy that person makes [post-birth energy] and is housed in the Heart. It is the most refined substance and is exceptionally important in the treatment of fertility.)[11, 12] Habits are worn, like monks' robes. We live within our habits, but we are also inhabited by them. It is possible to change habits but it takes work, a clear purpose and discipline, that is, to be a disciple to oneself. The amount of work required will relate to the depth that the habit has been ingrained.

Diet is about choosing the right foods to eat, when to eat them and how to eat them. Rushing food leads to its own problems and is perhaps a reflection of the type of food that is eaten.

WHEN TO EAT

TCM has long held the view that different organs and organ systems fluctuate in energy states. When it comes to diet, TCM understands that in humans the stomach is strongest early in the day. As the day lengthens, so the stomach becomes less strong and is weakest at night. Eating a healthy breakfast has been found to have a positive influence on cardiovascular health. Not eating breakfast, on the other hand, may significantly increase the potential to develop cardiovascular disease.[13]

Insulin secretion responds to a circadian rhythm. It is greatest between 6am and midday, and lowest at midnight, corresponding with the TCM view, and reflecting the relationship between the shift in glucose tolerance from breakfast time to dinner. Eating the largest meal of the day at night is unhealthy in many ways. People who work at night tend to higher BMIs and are at a significantly greater risk of developing diabetes.[14, 15, 16]

Really, our diet should start with a large breakfast, followed by a medium lunch and a light supper.

WHAT TO EAT

Insulin spikes should be avoided. Insulin is an excellent homeostatic energy storage hormone. It regulates energy by enabling cells to absorb glucose from the blood. In general, an increase in glucose is detected by the pancreas, which causes insulin to be secreted and freely available energy to be stored away. Whilst it's true that the spleen loves a sweet taste, too much sweetness will cause problems.

Choosing to eat something too sweet and/or processed in the morning can cause an insulin spike. The sweet, easily digestible food floods the system with freely available energy. The pancreas responds to this sudden increase in glucose by increasing secretion of insulin – bearing in mind that the morning is when we see a natural increase in insulin secretion, the pancreas essentially overcompensates. So, not only is the energy-dense food consumed quickly, but insulin stores away more glucose than normal, leading to a deficit of freely available energy which is signalled as hunger.

If a sweet breakfast happens very rarely, it's probably OK. But if a sweet breakfast is habitual, then it's going to be a problem. Perpetual hypersecretion of insulin will eventuate in a range of medical conditions. After consuming energy-dense food the initial hunger abates. However, it's easily digestible, easily used, and early in the habit easily stored. So, after the initial rush, hunger is once again experienced. Hunger abatement following sweet food consumption is usually managed by eating more sweet foods. A craving for energy-dense foods – fats and sugars – is very common now, and although the concept is still controversial, more than ever before we are now looking at a very large proportion in the Western world with an addiction to sugar.

Persistently managing life by consistently consuming too much energy-dense food in the form of highly processed, sweet foods will eventuate in a range of serious and potentially life-threatening medical conditions that will compromise fertility.

The US Central Intelligence Agency (CIA) has published a 2008 comparison of obesity levels by country. Of 191 countries, the United States came 19th, with a recorded obesity level of 33 per cent. The UK was 43rd with almost 27 per cent of its population registered as obese. Canada came 48th with just over 26 per cent. The populations of The Netherlands, Sweden, Denmark, France and Switzerland ranged in rank order, from 103rd (The Netherlands) to 111th (Switzerland), with the Netherlands recording obesity in almost 19 per cent of its population, and Switzerland recording obesity in 17.5 per cent of its population.[17]

These figures suggest that our fellow Europeans are doing something that promotes health. Types of diets may have something to do with this or the data may be interpreted more holistically as part of lifestyle. The Nordic diet is rich in oily fish, food stuffs that are full of Omega 3. The Mediterranean diet is also thought to be healthy, and Italy is 97th in the CIA world fact sheet of obesity.

8

Take Back Control Part 2

Fertility Antioxidants, Endocrine Disrupting Compounds, Epigenetics

ROS are free radicals. In low doses they are important contributory factors in reproductive function and successful fertility. However, when oxidative stress occurs, ROS are elevated beyond the total antioxidant capacity to regulate them and are toxic. Oxidative stress negatively affects fertility.

Antioxidants are molecules that regulate levels of both ROS and RNS. They provide a defence system in several ways: by donating an electron and thereby breaking the chain of molecular destruction that free radicals cause; by clearing them out altogether; and by repairing the damage caused.

There are two types of antioxidant systems: enzymatic and non-enzymatic antioxidants. Enzymatic antioxidants are endogenous, generated within the body, and rely on the way we nurture ourselves. For instance in humans, superoxide dismutases rely on copper, zinc and manganese, whereas the tremendously important enzymatic antioxidant glutathione relies on selenium. Thioredoxin system, also exceptionally important (in mice genetically mutated to be thioredoxin silent, four-cell embryonic failure occurs), in part also relies on selenium. Where stress has occurred (or even where stress hasn't in the case of selenium) supplementation of these minerals is available through the exogenous system. Exogenous antioxidants are known as synthetic antioxidants. The enzymatic system relies on exogenous antioxidants, both for supplementation where necessary, and to sustain optimal function of the antioxidant network.[1, 2, 3] Listed below are details of some key exogenous antioxidants and, because of its importance, glutathione.

Glutathione

This small endogenous antioxidant is an intercellular protein, is produced by all cells and with its wide and varied range of functions is often singled out as the most important antioxidant of all.

Glutathione (GSH) is a self-perpetuating molecule. It is formed by a synthesis of cysteine, glycine and part of the glutamate carboxyl group. Like other antioxidants it makes unstable molecules (free radicals) stable by donating an electron to an unstable molecule. A free radical seeks stability by 'stealing' an electron from a stable molecule, which then becomes reactive and 'steals' an electron from another stable molecule, and so the reaction chain continues.

The electron transfer causes stability in the free radical, and a radicalisation of the GSH molecule. But, there are many other reactive GSH molecules nearby with which the newly formed unstable molecule can bond. In so doing, the pair become a new molecule, glutathione disulfide (GSSG). Through a series of reactions GSSG is broken down into two antioxidant GSH molecules.

In general, there is considerably more GSH than GSSG. The ratio is often used to indicate the relative oxidative stress of an individual.

Recent research extols the value of GSH, now often thought of as the emperor of antioxidants. Both vitamins C and E are recycled by GSH;[4] it is an effective molecule in the inhibition of heavy metal poisoning,[5] carrying mercury and other heavy metals from the body whilst regulating lymphocytes, cytokines, T and NK cells; it is a metabolic invigorator, synthesiser and healer in many systems including the immune and nervous systems; and is absolutely vital in the production of iron.[6]

In addition to its role as an antioxidant, the existence of GSH receptors and physiological responses suggests the possibility that it may be a signalling compound in the neuroendocrine corpus. That GSH is regulated in a different way in early embryos and that an oxidative stress glutathionic protective system is established in early life suggest that GSH modulates embryo development. It is perhaps unsurprising then that in some circumstances a deficiency of GSH may be one of the causes in embryo pathogenesis.[7, 8]

Exogenous antioxidants

Vitamin C

Vitamin C is a very important antioxidant to have in your health chest. The Nobel Prize winner Linus Pauling advocated massive doses of vitamin C administered every day. This vitamin, ascorbic acid, is a preventative compound, inhibiting the damage caused by free radicals, such as degeneration of lipids (lipid peroxidation).

Lipids are hydrophobic compounds derived from fatty acids. In fact, many commentators consider the term 'lipid' synonymous with 'fatty acid' although international consensus on this term is quite unspecific. Fat, wax and oils are also often referred to as lipids. Vitamin E (tocopherol) is classed as a lipid.

Lipids comprise a long carbon chain which is either saturated or unsaturated. Here, saturation refers to a lipid compound replete with hydrogen, whereas unsaturated fatty acids are not, and due to their structure are able to pick up hydrogen atoms. So, saturation refers to the proportion of hydrogen and carbon; the more hydrogen than carbon, the more saturated the fat is. Saturated fats are usually solid at room temperature.

Unsaturated fat is also differentiated into either polyunsaturated or monounsaturated fat. Olive oil is a monounsaturated fat and has only one double-bonded carbon molecule. The essential fatty acid linoleic acid, found in Omega 6 oil, is a polyunsaturated fat because it has more than one double-bonded carbon in the chain.

ROS are a natural life event, an endogenous by-product of mitochondrial respiration (amongst other causes). Often, the production of ROS outweighs the total antioxidant capacity, leading to oxidative stress. This causes damage to lipids and proteins. An example of the danger is the oxidation of low-density lipoprotein (LDL, also known as bad cholesterol) by ROS (and potentially other biochemicals), which eventually causes atherosclerosis. LDL is derived from very-low-density lipoprotein (vLDL). There appears to be a relationship between polycystic ovarian syndrome and elevated ROS, and women with PCOS appear to be at a much greater risk of increased vLDL levels.[9, 10]

Other than its antioxidant properties, vitamin C is also an important factor in the creation of collagen, and for hormones. In women, it is abundant in the ovaries, and is also present in the pituitary. It appears to be required for hormone synthesis, and responds to fluctuations in gonadotropin secretory patterns and urinary levels of vitamin C fluctuating in accordance with gonadotropic changes. This may be a natural response to its regulatory effect on LH. It also appears to be associated with luteal phase defect. A trial published in 2003 evaluated the effect of ascorbic acid on patients suffering from luteal phase defect (LPD). Following treatment, both oestrogen and serum progesterone levels increased. Moreover, a significantly higher pregnancy rate was observed in the treatment group.[11]

Vitamin B

Oxidative stress may occur when vitamin B6 is deficient. When there is sufficient B6, it helps to regulate hormones and extend the luteal phase and seems to improve cervical mucus. Vitamin B12 also appears to help regulate the menstrual cycle, and when it is taken with calcium it may help to control cortisol and regulate hormonal expression. Low levels of vitamin B6 and B12 (and folic acid) are associated with the condition that precedes the onset of stroke.

Folic acid (folate) is one of the vitamin B complex (vitamin B9) and because our species cannot synthesise it, folate is an essential substance. It is involved in DNA synthesis and repair, in the production or red blood cells and healthy blood, and for fertility it is especially important due to its enhancement of cell division and cell growth. The name is derived from 'folium', the Latin for 'leaf', which provides an indication of the dietary source of this substance. It's probably impossible to get the recommended dose from leafy greens however. It's also best to remain within the recommended limits, since too much appears to be implicated as a causative cancer factor.

Vitamin D (cholecalciferol, abbreviated to calciferol)

How many times have you heard of people going on holiday and falling pregnant? Is it just that a holiday improves mood, stress is released, enjoyment thrives? It could also be that vitamin D is increased. Sunlight converts sterols present on the skin to form vitamin D, although the rate of conversion is very much dependent on skin type; darker skin requires a greater amount of ultraviolet exposure. Other sources of vitamin D include oils from fish and cod liver oil, eggs and milk.

Although calciferol is termed a vitamin, in fact it behaves like a hormone, looks like a hormone and should be considered a hormone. It is created endogenously (although dietary supplementation is often required), and once converted becomes hormonally active, and behaves like other sterol hormones. It is known to be a regulator of calcium and phosphorus, and is directly involved in mineral absorption, particularly calcium absorption in the intestines. Importantly, it appears that there is a significant correspondence between low levels of vitamin d and autoimmune diseases, and particularly autoimmune diseases affecting the thyroid.[12]

Recently, evidence has begun to generate a broader picture of the effects of vitamin D. It is present in most cells in the body and is implicated in cellular growth and differentiation, regulation of the immune system and the hormonal milieu, inhibition of cancer, and hypertension, and contributes to the prevention of osteoporosis. Low levels of vitamin D are associated with obesity and endocrine disturbances. From a fertility point of view, both male and female fertility may be compromised by inappropriate levels of vitamin D. In women, elevated vitamin D is implicated in endometriosis, whereas deficient vitamin D levels are implicated in PCOS, infertility and poor IVF success rates. Many patients appear to have significantly low levels of calciferol and a regular blood test should be sought.

Vitamin E

Vitamin E (tocopherol) is another important molecule to combat oxidative stress, and its benefits are many. Once again, however, the evidence provides a divergent picture; in some studies, vitamin E seems to help with a variety of conditions; in others, it appears to make no difference. The areas that are most commonly investigated are heart, respiration and mental health, macular degeneration and the reproductive cycle.

When vitamin E stabilises a free radical, it also becomes destabilised. This process is reversed by the actions of several other antioxidants, including vitamin C.

Vitamin E is involved in the production of prostaglandins. Prostaglandins are involved in the production of prolactin. Both prostaglandins and prolactin are involved in premenstrual syndrome.

WHAT ARE PROSTAGLANDINS?

Prostaglandins are a family of organic molecules, and one of the sub-families belonging to the eicosanoid group (derived from the Greek *eikosa*, meaning 'twenty', *eidos*, meaning 'form', and *noic*, which is the suffix applied to names of fatty acids (combined from *ane* and *ioc*). They were discovered independently by two scientists, Ulf von Euler and M.W. Goldblatt, in 1935. Von Euler originally thought they were made in the prostate gland, hence the name. However, it is now known that prostaglandins are synthesised in almost every cell, have a short life span and only travel very short distances. They are therefore paracrine and autocrine messengers and act to maintain local homeostasis. Their effect is mediated by their receptors and they are powerful vasoactive molecules, causing either dilation or constriction of smooth muscle.

In terms of disease, perhaps the most significant attribute of prostaglandins is their role in the inflammatory response. Inflammation is essentially a branch of the immune system and is involved in many disease processes including stroke, ateriosclerosis, cardiovascular disease including atherosclerosis, and cancer. Prostaglandin production is mobilised immediately in response to inflammation by catalysis of the oxadising agent, hydrogen peroxide (because of the nature of its bond, H_2O_2 readily donates the extra oxygen atom), by cyclooxygenases (COXs) in either of its forms. Both COX-1 and COX-2 are required for normal fertility, pregnancy and labour, and can generate secretion of organic compounds necessary for regulatory functions and homeostasis. Both can also generate prostanoid secretion involved in the inflammatory response. However, COX-2 is the enzyme associated with the latter tendency.

COX-1 and COX-2 synthesise PGH2, which in turn leads to the production of the prostaglandins PGD2, PGE2 and PGF2.

Prostaglandins are intimately involved across the range of inflammatory symptoms. For the patient, probably the most noticeable is the production of inflammation and pain, although other effects occur including reduction in oxygen flow, muscle contraction/vasodilation and immune enhancement.

Endometriosis, the condition where endometrial tissue becomes attached to tissue external to the uterus, is also associated with production and elevated secretion of prostaglandins. Endometriotic tissue is the site of inflammation. Growing where it should not be growing will cause inflammation; displacing organs by pulling them out of place will cause inflammation; interfering with fimbriae, interfering with the ovaries and ovarian function, even the uterus, will cause inflammation.

Women with endometriosis suffer from pelvic pain, often chronic, dysmenorrhoea (that is, painful periods) and dyspareunia (painful sexual intercourse). Although the cause of endometriosis is unknown, one of the prostaglandin family, PGE2, is known to be the dominating prostaglandin in endometriosis.

Eicosanoids are lipids, and in the main are derived from arachidonic acid (from *arachos*, meaning 'legume'), the polyunsaturated Omega-6 fatty acid. Being an eicosatetraenoic acid (ETA), the structure of arachidonic acid includes a straight 20-carbon chain.

Arachidonic acid is an Omega-6 fatty acid, and although not essential (there are only two essential fatty acids) it can become essential when linoleic acid is insufficient. Whilst it can be freely available it is mostly stored within the cell membrane in phospholipids, to be released by receptor-triggered hydrolysis. Once released from its phospholipid latency, it will be converted by the action of either one of two synthases: COX or lipoxygenase. Its ultimate functional fate will depend on whichever synthase has been involved in the conversion. Cyclooxygenase (COX) is the synthase responsible for the creation of a group of eicosanoid families, the prostanoids, of which the prostaglandins are one.

Arachidonic acid tends to produce pro-inflammatory molecules such as prostanoids, which increase production of pro-inflammatory cytokines associated with chronic inflammatory diseases.

Omega-3, on the other hand, comes from fish oils and is a monounsaturated fat. Other monounsaturated fats are derived from plant oils (olive oil for instance), some nuts and avacodos. Fish oils are the origin of the highly beneficial polyunsaturated fats such as eicosapentaenoic acid (EPA), a cardiovascular health promoter, and docosahexaenoic acid (DHA), thought to be very beneficial for memory and learning.

In addition to fish oils, egg yolks, red meats and offal are high in arachidonic acid. It is beneficial in small doses, but too much is bad for you. In fact, elevated insulin levels seem to cause greater secretion of arachidonic acid. It's worth considering whether there is a correlation between the (assumed) subsequent production and secretion of pro-inflammatory molecules such as prostaglandins and the pre-proinflammator ratio of elevated insulin. What is quite interesting is that prostaglandins have a significantly pronounced presence in endometriosis.

In terms of diet, the ratio of ararchidonic acid to other foods is really important. We know that weight appears to be significantly involved in successful fertility attempts and often people will be following a particular diet. Some diets advocate an absolute carbohydrate restriction, whereas others recommend high chicken or turkey or salmon diets, with significant carbohydrate restriction. As you may know, chicken and turkey (and even farmed salmon since in many cases the salmon have been fed corn) have a much higher ratio of arachidonic acid to protein than even beef.

Pharmaceuticals

Statins, used to treat arteriosclerosis, increase arachidonic acid, leading to cellular inflammation, which in turn increases resistance to insulin.

NSAIDS are essentially COX inhibitors. So, whilst cyclo-oxygenase is inhibited and therefore production of inflammators such as prostaglandins is also restricted, the total arachidonic acid count remains unchanged.

Supplements and foods that will restrict the damage done by consumption of arachidonic acid include monounsaturated fats derived from fish oils.

Selenium (Se)

Selenium is a potent antioxidant with wide-ranging effects on cellular function. Selenium is also the component of most of the forms of the antioxidant glutathione (GSH). This antioxidant is deeply involved in cellular integrity, cellular growth and cellular signalling. It is involved in the prevention of cancer, cardiovascular disease and endocrine function. It is also intrinsically involved in a protective capacity in thyroid hormone synthesis and metabolism. Deficiency in selenium is implicated in miscarriage, foetal growth restriction and preeclampsia. Selenium is therefore a very important fertility mineral.

The natural availability of selenium is derived from the growth of food on selenium-rich soil. Where selenium is deficient in soil, so will the food stuffs be. Selenium can be obtained from fish, poultry and eggs, and is exceptionally high in brazil nuts, which provide an excellent dietary supply of selenium.[13]

Zinc (Zn)

As with many nutritional supplements, scientific research is only just beginning, and the data on the properties of zinc are a reflection of this. Nevertheless, zinc is being established as another highly important fertility mineral and is known to be a requirement for healthy reproduction in both men and women. It is a required mineral for LH and FSH, and modulates protein synthesis in early pregnancy. Some reports suggest that zinc may be responsible for dysregulation of the menstrual cycle, miscarriage and problems associated with pregnancy, such as preeclampsia.

Zinc is also a potent antioxidant, and inhibits the damaging effects of ROS on DNA. As a co-factor for folic acid metabolism, a deficiency of zinc can lead to a deficiency in folic acid absorption, leading to a reduction in antioxidant capacity. It is also a co-factor in DNA transcription, which is deeply important in the maturation of germ cells. Zinc, then, is probably highly important for egg quality.

Beta-carotene

Very little work has been published on this compound. The little that has been done, however, does provide some insight into its potential effects. There is a high level of beta-carotene in the corpus luteum, from which the corpus luteum derives its yellow colour.[14] In animals, however, adequate levels of beta-carotene appear to improve both fertility and successful pregnancy.[15, 16]

Beta-carotene is a precursor of vitamin A. Vitamin A (also known as retinol) is known to be an important fertility compound in both men and women. Vitamin A deficiency (VAD) can lead to decreased reproductive capacity, at a meiotic level and at the embryogenesis level, and pregnancy failing before implantation. Where vitamin A levels are restored, so pregnancy seems to survive. If levels are raised too much though, vitamin A becomes lethal to the embryo.

Alpha lipoic acid

Alpha lipoic acid is a precursor to GSH and has been widely described as an antioxidant that is at least as potent as GSH. Like GSH it is an endogenous antioxidant and is both hydrophilic and lipophilic – so it achieves results by being both water (hydrophilic) and fat (lipophilic) soluble. This means that, like GSH, it can work with antioxidants of either breed. For example, both ascorbic acid, which is a water-soluble substance and lipophobic, and tocopherol (vitamin E), which is a fat-soluble substance and hydrophobic, are allied and can in fact be regenerated by lipoic acid. This substance is found in offal (particularly liver) and yeast.

The structure of lipoic acid means that it passes through the blood–brain barrier with relative ease, and so may be useful in inhibiting damage caused by oxidative stress in the brain. Some studies have found that people suffering from peripheral neuropathy had a significant reduction in their symptoms when taking lipoic acid. There is some evidence that it has some anti-aging properties, some of which are related to the visible effects of oxidative stress on the skin.

There have been some side effects reported when this substance has been taken, including skin rashes and headaches. It has also been found that lipoic acid can cause the excretion of heavy metals, as with GSH. Unlike GSH, however, lipoic acid has been found to carry heavy metals from the concentrated origin to other tissue (particularly the brain). This is a concern and it is reasonable to postulate that lipoic acid may be implicated in the rare condition insulin autoimmune syndrome, seen most commonly in Japan.

Lipoic acid is exceptionally important for blood sugar levels and cardiovascular health. It has far-reaching benefits for type 2 diabetes, helping to convert sugar, and people suffering from this disease and taking lipoic acid saw significant improvements in their sugar conversion, which was nearly twice as fast as those suffering from type 2 diabetes but not taking it.[17] Neuropathic symptoms derived from this condition have also been significantly improved.

Lipoic acid is roundly acclaimed as an antioxidant par excellence. In spite of this, at this time there has been very little work on the effects of this antioxidant on female fertility. Given that it is so versatile, and involved in so many systems that are both directly and indirectly involved in fertility, it cannot be long before we see a tranche of trials evaluating the effects of this compound on female reproduction.

Environment

Energy is formed from the food we eat and the air we breathe, so contaminated air will influence energy production, and maybe even the quality of energy (although we would require fairly sophisticated technology to measure the difference). Contaminated food will also influence energy production, and in this case it is much easier to measure good from bad energy.

That the environment can alter oocyte quality is evident. Consider ICSI and the consequences of that ART procedure. Consider that follicular development relies on blood flow and oxygen, the quality of which has been shown to influence oocyte competence. Or consider the effect of radiation.[18]

Endocrine disrupting compounds

The authors of the French study point out that there are a number of socio-economic factors that could be responsible for the results of their trial, and particularly reference EDCs as a potential cause.

Bisphenol A (BPA), a known endocrine disruptor, is now banned from use in baby bottles. However, both BPA and bisphenol S can leach into food and liquids through plastics when hot or scratched. This includes water bottles and other household products such as CDs, toys and reusable plastic implements. Canned food and other ubiquitous household containers (such as drinking containers) are often lined with a resin of which BPA is a component.

Other EDCs include dioxins (toxic emissions derived from manufacturing, burning waste – industrial or residential – cigarette smoke, pesticides which may be present in food in some cases, usually at a very low level), polychlorinated biphenyls, widely used in the US until 1977, and some pesticides. Another group of chemicals thought to be EDCs are phthalates, widely used in products for human consumption including many cosmetics, vinyl products and food packaging. The National Library of Medicine has developed a useful website resource that provides information on toxic substances, called Tox Town. The site reports that in 1999, their use in baby products such as teethers and pacifiers ceased as a result of pressure from the US Consumer Product Safety Commission.[19]

BPA is an oestrogen mimic. It can lead to functional and morphological changes in the reproductive systems of both women and men, and in any tissue relying on the endocrine system. Such is the scope of EDCs that it only requires a simple stretch of the imagination to apprehend how these products, ubiquitous in our lives, could interrupt key processes in fertility and in the development of reproductive systems. Evidence on this subject has begun to accumulate.[20, 21]

Given their ubiquity in our society, it is unsurprising that EDCs have been found in follicular fluid. The presence of EDCs in follicular fluid is linked to decreased fertilisation rate. This is interpreted to be a reflection of egg quality: that the EDCs have negatively affected the egg. If the quality of the egg is compromised then it's likely that embryo development will also be compromised, since the quality of the embryo relies on the quality of both sperm and egg.[22]

The effect of EDCs on descendants appears to depend on age. Whilst adult exposure will affect the adult with usual recovery from illness and functional impairment, exposure of the embryo to EDCs during the pre-implantation period will not only permanently affect the offspring, but also their descendents. Intrauterine exposure to EDCs at the time of embryonic ovarian development can alter the reproductive organs, causing infertility. The effects of EDCs on ovarian development are surely going to cause far-reaching and most likely transgenerational effects in offspring.

In fact, in 2009, the Endocrine Society issued a Scientific Statement which presented evidence that 'endocrine disruptors have effects on male and female reproduction, breast development and cancer, prostate cancer, neuroendocrinology, thyroid, metabolism and obesity, and cardiovascular endocrinology'. The Endocrine Society further claim that:

> EDCs involve divergent pathways including (but not limited to) oestrogenic, antiandrogenic, thyroid, peroxisome proliferator activated receptor y, retinoid and actions through other nuclear receptors; steroidogenic enzymes; neurotransmitter receptors and systems; and many other pathways that are highly conserved in wildlife and humans.[23]

To say this is a little worrying is truly an understatement. The numbers of pathways these chemicals are involved in, the numbers of systems those pathways are involved in, and the number of conditions that the use of EDCs most likely either cause or are causative factors in is extremely worrying. Questions immediately spring to mind: since EDCs influence the endocrine system, which is known to influence our emotions, to what extent are EDCs influencing our emotions? To what extent is the current epidemic of obesity a result of the use of EDCs? Or other modern epidemics? How extensive are the effects of EDCs in endocrine systems that are already matured? What is the extent of EDCs in the corruption of endocrine systems that are still in the early stages of maturing?

Endocrine disrupting compounds and male fertility

Although this book is about female fertility, EDCs have been shown to affect both sexes.

The quality of semen has been found to be a reasonable reflection of a man's life span.[24] I am surprised that insurers haven't yet started using it. If male gonadofunction is a reflection of longevitiy, then it's probable that a similar indication can be derived from female gonadofunction. In terms of fertility, ultimately the fertilisation of the egg will be from a sperm. ICSI does lead to increased chances of foetal problems, so it's worth taking a brief look at what's happening to male fertility.

It looks concerning and the decline in male fertility is often reported in the press in terms of an epidemic. Such reports do not include the worrying rise in testicular cancer, particularly in Canada where the rate has increased by 50 per cent in the last 25 years.[25–32]

A study published in 2009 from Denmark evaluated the semen analyses of 43,277 men presenting for infertility treatment and compared the results to the Danish population. The investigators found that as sperm quantity and quality increased, so did life expectancy in a manner that was dose dependent; men with healthy sperm up to a threshold of 40 million/ml were likely to have a decreased early mortality rate of 43 per cent. The results suggest that early mortality increases as sperm quantity and quality (motility and morphology) decreases, and the chances of early mortality increase in a dose dependent manner. The authors concluded that the resultant decrease could not be attributable to social factors alone.[33]

In France, a study concluded that in the last 17 years the average total sperm count has dropped by just over 32 per cent, and the number of healthy sperm has also dropped by almost a third. While it is true that neither the drop in the average total sperm count, nor the drop in the numbers of healthy sperm mean that the men were infertile, if the conclusions and the interpretations from the Danish study are correct, there has been a 30 per cent increase in the chances of an early death in French men in less than 20 years.[34]

Epigenetics

It appears that EDCs are not thought to directly cause genetic mutations. However, EDCs do have the capacity to cause changes in the epigenome.

Genetics (from the Greek *genesis*, meaning 'origin') is the study and science of heredity and variation of heredity in organisms, and is derived from Gregor Mendel's (1822–1884) work, although later researchers independently replicated his work. Mendel's theory of genetics was synthesised with Darwin's theory of natural selection in the twentieth century to form the current evolutionary theory.

Epigenetics (from the Greek *epi*, meaning 'on top of' or 'in addition to'), on the other hand, is the theory of hereditable change that is caused by systems other than changes in the DNA sequence. Epigenetics also refers to functional changes to the genome. Functional and hereditable changes of the genome that occur above the DNA sequence include the processes of methylation and histone modification.

The genome (from the German *gen*, derived from 'gene', and 'om', derived from the German *Chromosom*) is the consistent, essentially static record of genetic information in cells across the entire DNA sequence and genes.

An epigenome is a record of the functional changes to DNA. The epigenome also controls the functional expression of genes and, in this case, the environment that influences primordial germ cells. Primordial germ cells arise in the embryo at a very early stage and migrate to the gonads. They're present in both males and females. In the ovary, they become oocytes at the end of the first trimester.

The term epigenetics is derived from Conrad Waddington (1905–1975), a developmental biologist. It can be thought of and is often described as a form of 'soft inheritance' promulgated by Lamarckians, derived from the work of Jean Baptiste Lamarck (1744–1829), *Philosphie Zoologique* (1809), although its core is fundamentally different to the mechanisms espoused by Larmarck.

The concept of epigenetics theorises that environment modulates genetics: that non-genetic factors can modify functions of DNA, which can be transferred down the ancestral line (transgenerational epigenetics). So evolution may be driven by factors not relating directly to natural selection. An example of this is the domestication of wolves to produce dogs, a series of events that occurred around 15,000 years ago. To test epigenetic evolution, a recent attempt was made by Dmitry Belyaev to domesticate silver foxes. Using training and selection, Belyaev managed to domesticate a group of silver foxes within 20 years of breeding, ten times faster than species mutation through natural selection.[35, 36, 37]

Hard inheritance theorises that evolution is fixed, that DNA is held static by histone. It originates in the theories developed by Darwin and Mendel and which represent the backbone of *Evolution: The Modern Synthesis*, which states that the DNA of an embryo will not be influenced by the experience of its parents.[38]

In embryo development, the epigenome of the embryo goes through a process of reprogramming, that is, erasing the epigenetic information, or chemical tags or marks, left on the DNA in primordial germ cells from each parental genetic line. 'Reprogramming' is the process of DNA methylation, where genes from both parents are marked and rendered inactive. DNA methylation is a one-way ticket, the biochemical equivalent of Lethe, the river of forgetfulness in ancient Greek legend. As a result of the methylation process, the experience of parental past attached to genetic material is obliterated. Or is supposed to be. Recent research has found that DNA methylation is incomplete in some cases, to ensure that hereditable genes are regulated, for instance, and this latter process is an epigenetic phenomenon called genomic imprinting.

DNA doesn't change, except in very rare circumstances. DNA methylation, however, can be modulated, and the novel field of nutritional epigenetics is beginning to bear fruit.

The Barker Hypothesis of 1995 correlates the way a baby grows in the womb with maternal nutrition and the nourishment of the foetus, and low birth weight and early infant nourishment with adult metabolic disease.[39]

Initially, Professor Barker looked at death rates due to CHD in the UK. He found that regions with high death rates from CHD correlated with regions with high infant mortality rates from 70 years before. The question he then asked was whether the pregnancy of the mothers of the surviving infants in those regions had suffered hardship. The results of this initial work demonstrated that low birth weight seems to predict adult onset of CHD. It also proved to be the genesis of the 'Thrifty Phenotype' hypothesis (sometimes called the Barker Hypothesis); that the nutritional status of the mother will form the basis for the adult health of the foetus she is carrying.

Many other research studies have since been undertaken to correlate foetal and infant nutrition with adult metabolic disease. Probably one of the most significant in terms of the developmental origins of disease is the study on the World War II Dutch Famine.

The Dutch Famine occurred during the winter of 1944/1945 when the Nazis blockaded the transport of food and fuel into a region in the Netherlands. Four and a half million million people were affected. Although most survived, calorific restriction became extremely severe. Even with extensive rationing, food stocks virtually disappeared. By November, meat ceased to be available at all, and by April the surviving population were eking out an existence on 400g of bread, 1kg of potatoes and less than a teaspoonful of vegetable oil per week.[40] Pregnant women who lived through this event gave birth to children born with a normal birth weight, on average, but babies who suffered maternal malnutrition during early gestation seemed to have a predisposition to develop CHD as adults.[41]

Although the average birth weight was normal for offspring of the survivors, what was unexpected was that the offspring of those infants, grown to adulthood and with an unrestricted diet, gave birth to infants with low birth weight and a predisposition to a range of metabolic diseases in adulthood.[42, 43, 44, 45] The affects of maternal nutrition are transgenerational.[46]

Essentially, that a trait should evolve and be passed on generationally suggests a phenomenon called 'programming', outlined in a paper by Hendrina Boo and Jane Harding (2006).[47] Programming can involve mechanisms such as foetal nourishment, where under- or over-nourishment can cause alterations in normal foetal development. A further mechanism relates to elevated stress hormones, such as cortisol. Mechanisms such as these can cause the foetus to adapt in order to survive. Often, environmental events that trigger these mechanisms pass relatively quickly and so the adaptations can be reversible. However, if the events persist, the foetal response will cause adaptations that are irreversible. An example of an environmental event at a particular time during gestation causing irreversible deviation of the normal evolution of the foetus is seen in foetal alcohol syndrome.

Irreversible adaptations will involve changes at the genetic level. Given what is currently known, the appropriate theory to begin to address these phenomena is the epigenetic/soft inheritance corps. The process of methylation, that is remethylation and demethylation of certain maternal and paternal genes, is thought to particularly influence embryonic growth and development.[48] Methylation is modulated in part by diet. In both mouse and rat models, diets deficient in methyl donors caused dysregulation of the methylation process. Methyl donors include substances such as vitamin B12 (folate), garlic and onions, and certain phytoestrogens derived from soy.

9 Evidence

Placebo, Evidence, Narrative

> It is important to distinguish the very respectable, conscious use of placebos. The effect of placebos has been shown by randomised controlled trials to be very large. Their use in the correct place is to be encouraged. What is inefficient is the use of relatively expensive drugs as placebos.[1]

The use of the word 'placebo' in medicine most likely derives from one of the Psalms (originally Psalm 116) from the Catholic ritual, the Office of the Vespers of the Dead.

It is known that the Office of the Vespers of the Dead acquired its current form during the eighth century (at the behest of Pope Gregory III[2]) but originates at the very least from the seventh century. As in later centuries it was sung at funerals on behalf of a particular soul, and from 735 on All Souls' Day on behalf of all souls in purgatory.

The origins of the word placebo in the Office of Vespers of the Dead, however, is derived from St Jerome's translation of the Bible into Latin during the fourth century. The Hebrew word 'ethalech', meaning 'I will walk with' or 'be in step with', was replaced with the Latin word 'placebo', meaning 'I shall please'.

The modern concept of 'placebo' probably involves the phenomenon of 'placebo singers' whose origins are derived mostly from France in the Middle Ages. It was the custom for wealthy families to provide feasts in honour of their departed. Placebo singers, people either distantly related or entirely unrelated to the family, would attend the funerals to partake of the largesse, and would begin their petition by singing from the 'Placebo' from the Vespers.

The placebo effect

The placebo effect has been elicited for a long time. Its use in medical terminology began in the late eighteenth century and was understood as 'a medicine given more to please than to benefit the patient'.[3]

Three centuries ago placebo medicine was commonplace, and understood as part of the medical corpus (although Jefferson recorded it as a 'pious fraud').[4] Two centuries ago, placebo was understood as a necessary deceit practised by the doctor on the patient to help the patient feel better, and many products said to be a 'cure-all' were derived simply from sugar. In the US, even up until 1963 pharmaceutical companies needed only to prove the safety of the product, not any medical efficacy. Recently, a Parliamentary Commission evaluating the use of homeopathy in the NHS concluded that on the balance of evidence, homeopathy should be considered a placebo, and that the prescription of a placebo 'usually relies on some degree of deception'.[5] At some point in history the concept of placebo moved from something involving a spiritual approach in medicine to something involving deceit.

A placebo can be a substance or treatment that is traditionally considered to have no medical effect (and now stated as effects unkown) and yet provided for a patient's relief. However, many research studies have now found that even where a patient is told that the substance they are going to take is a placebo, the placebo can produce a postitive effect. The placebo effect is also thought to be involved in almost every therapeutic technique.

Is the placebo effect the same as spontaneous regression?

In distinction to spontaneous remission, which is defined as the complete disappearance of the disease, spontaneous regression is defined as the decrease of disease in the absence of any previous treatment, or treatment with a therapy that is thought to be unable to exert a significant influence on neoplastic disease, so could spontaneous regression be a form of placebo?[6, 7, 8, 9] Reports of it are extant in almost every type of human cancer. In one report incidence of spontaneous regression in breast cancer was as much as 22 per cent.[10]

The incidence of spontaneous regression in cancer is also often correlated with an acute infectious disease. An acute infectious disease will involve the inflammatory/immune response. Although the exact mechanism is yet to be determined, an analysis published in 2001 demonstrated that hyperthermic reaction induced by acute infectious disease or pyrogenic substances may promote a 'spontaneous regression' of disease. It is also suggested that the sufferance of such an infectious disease in children may protect them against future cancer.[11]

The relationship between an acute infectious disease and the mobilisation of an acute inflammatory response to treat cancer was exploited in the late nineteenth and early twentieth centuries by William Coley, whose remedy Coley's Toxins was used in treating many forms of cancer. A comparative analysis between Coley's Toxins and radiotherapy demonstrated that the Toxins were as effective as radiotherapy cancer treatments until the early 1980s.[12] Although it was a novel approach, the induction of a feverish state to cure cancer or cancer-like symptoms was also used in the very ancient past.[13]

Induction of the inflammatory/immune response is also suggested to be the mechanism by which the uterine scratch, also known as the pipelle, may work in improving pregnancy rates. By scratching the uterus, inflammatory and immune biochemicals are secreted, which may either influence the appositing blastocyst, or modulate the endometrium and uterine environment, or both.

So incidences of spontaneous regression may actually have a cause and may not be due to a placebo effect after all. However, many suggest that the placebo effect is the very basis of healing.

The placebo effect is shown to increase the effect of medicine, and the effect varies between patients, from around 30 per cent to over 60 per cent.[14, 15] Cure rates of 75 per cent and even 100 per cent have also been reported.[16] The effect increases according to condition; conditions that appear to relate to an emotional/mental attitude or aspect appear to respond better to the placebo effect than conditions that are purely physical. Examples of the two types of conditions include conditions classed as mental/emotional such as depression, and cardiovascular conditions such as high blood pressure.

A positive outlook influences health. Although there is a lively debate between classical conditioning and expectancy, expectancy and belief are thought to be a potential pathway through which the placebo effect works. Since this is the case, when given a sugar pill, both positive and negative outcomes of the 'treatment' can be determined by the information the trial subject is given.[17] Since expectancy and belief play a part in the outcome of a medical intervention, an optimistic approach should improve a patient's chances following a medical diagnosis. Several studies have shown just that, including significantly increased life expectancy, increased immunity, and increased chances of successful IVF outcome. Optimism may even provide a predictor for a woman's biological response in an IVF cycle.[18, 19, 20]

In fact, so great is the power of the placebo effect, it is remarkable that this medical adjunct has not been truly investigated. Research being undertaken now is beginning to find pathways.

At the Harvard Medical School, the Program in Placebo Studies & Therapeutic Encounter is developing a set of criteria that delineates, at least in part, a method to elicit the placebo effect. These criteria include empathy, duration of interaction between the doctor and patient, and positivity. In a recent study, it appears that increasing factors known to be associated in the mobilisation of placebo effect increase its effectiveness. When factors involved in the placebo effect are increased, so the effectiveness of the treatment is increased and so the scientists conclude that the placebo effect is dose dependent.[21]

Brain imaging studies are also trying to map out changes in brain activity. Studying the effect of placebo-induced anaethesia, results of brain imaging are showing activity changes in areas that are thought to be associated with discomfort or motivation to change, anticipation and perception, all of which appear to be involved in the placebo effect.[22, 23]

A word on evidence

Evidence-based medicine (EBM) is derived from clinical epidemiology. The word itself comprises the Greek words *epi*, *demos* ('people') and *logos* ('study'). It is the study of patterns and causes of disease and treatments, and has led to further development in medicine called evidence-based practice, or evidence-based healthcare.

The evolution of EBM extends back many centuries. One of its applications in modern medicine is the evaluation of the efficacy of a treatment based on the results of a single or a number of clinical trials. The strength of a clinical trial is in turn based on its design. There are quite a few methodologies for trial designs. In both the UK and the US, the gold standard is the triple blind, placebo controlled, randomised controlled trial (RCT). This combination of blinding and randomisation is effective because it obviates bias in both the treater and the treated. Even down to the provision of a pill, the person providing the pill may imply that the pill may have or may not have a beneficial effect. By randomising the trial, all the participants – the treaters, the treated and the evaluators – remain blind to who received treatment. In this way, any bias that may influence the result of the trial should be avoided.

The BMJ recently published an article entitled 'What conclusions has *Clinical Evidence* drawn about what works, what doesn't based on randomised controlled trial evidence?'[24] The article identifies the difficulty in categorising treatments: for example, a treatment might have been found to be beneficial in the treatment of one condition, but will have no benefit in another. This is similar to the use of an acupuncture point prescription to induce ovulation in women suffering from oligo/anovulation due to polycystic ovarian syndrome and to use the same point prescription to try to induce labour.[25]

Of the three thousand WM treatments evaluated and reported in the *BMJ* article, 3 per cent are likely to be ineffective or harmful, in 7 per cent there is a trade off between benefits and harms, 5 per cent have been shown to have no benefit, 11 per cent have been found to be clinically effective, 24 per cent are likely to be beneficial, and 50 per cent of treatments are of unknown effectiveness, meaning there is no evidence concerning these treatments.

The fact that in many cases research trials have not been undertaken is perhaps unsurprising. Research trials cost money and are expensive. Further, it does not mean that those therapeutic interventions not backed by research should be considered ineffective. EBM is defined as 'the conscientious, explicit and judicious use of current best evidence in making decisions about the care of individual patients'[26] devised as a guide to medical practitioners, to be used alongside experience acquired in clinical practice, and not to supplant it.[27]

That EBM could supplant clinical experience as the prime criteria in patient management, treatment and discharge is still argued, and in some cases vociferously. There are several charges laid against EBM; that it does not meet its own empirical tests of efficacy, and that it is not therefore evidence based,[28, 29] that it erodes the art of medicine,[30] that it is a microfascism,[31] that it will eventually extinguish the patient, to name a few. The latter perspective, from medical humanists, argues that EBM 'strips patients of their stories and the meaning of their experience, reducing them to passive recipients of doctor-centred communications',[32] an argument not limited to social scientists but also some from a medical backgound.[33]

The medical humanist perspective is countered in part by a view which suggests that EBM empowers patients so that a patient is a 'rational choice actor'.[34] By delivering information about the best clinical evidence available, derived from well-designed, operationalised and conducted research trials to patients, patients are better able to balance the risk–benefit ratio of the treatments available.[35] Aside from other points regarding evidence and quality of evidence, many point out that this new method of clinical communication presents new demands to the patient and unfortunately doesn't deal with the problem of patient narrative.

The problems with EBM, voiced more than a decade ago, are still with us, and have still not been answered.

Acupuncture is a highly researched therapy. In 2011, Ji Sheng Han and Yuh-Shan Ho published a bibliometric analysis in *Neuroscience and Biobehavourial Reviews* entitled 'Global trends and performances of acupuncture research', and evaluated the number of trials and categories from 1991 to 2009 published in English. Overall they found 6004 publications over the 19 years. The US was the main producer of research, followed closely by China, which in 2009 overtook the US in the production of research. The UK ranked fourth, after South Korea.[36] However, with a population of 1.2 billion, eight hundred million of whom are Mandarin speakers, it is very unlikely that the majority of research papers from China will ever be published in English.

As with many modern researchers, the authors mention the difficulty in establishing a placebo effect, and since the placebo effect is involved in the outcome of all medical treatments, evaluating an acupuncture point prescription in a controlled trial really does require a control for placebo.

Acupuncture is well established as an effective treatment for pain. Modulation of opioids in the central nervous system (CNS) appears to be one of the mechanisms involved in the effectiveness of the acupuncture treatments. Several trials have evaluated the effect of acupuncture treatments against 'sham' acupuncture. Although generally both are more effective than having no treatment, in some cases the control arm (sham acupuncture) may be found to be as effective as the intervention arm acupuncture and in some cases more effective.[37, 38] Is this because of the acupuncture treatments, or because of a placebo effect, or both?

Often, the evaluation of an acupuncture treatment by a clinical trial seems to be similar to the research evaluation of a pill and, in fact, the results are usually proclaimed by the media in the same way as a drugs trial. But acupuncture is a procedure, not a pill. A trial to evaluate an acupuncture treatment of a particular condition is not an evaluation of the entire therapy in that treatment of that particular condition. If it were, then it would be like saying a trial to evaluate a surgical technique is an evaluation of the entire discipline of surgery. Since neither surgery nor acupuncture are pills, a trial to evaluate either of these disciplines requires very careful planning indeed.

Often, a trial of the effect of acupuncture in the treatment of a condition is devised to determine the clinical efficacy of a point prescription, the needle technique and trial methodology. Secondary points may also reflect the environment that the trial participant, the subject, will be placed in during the trial.

The complexity of interactions in the human body is beyond imagining. Since acupuncture has been shown to modulate a range of neurotransmitters, it is very difficult to imagine an effective placebo using an acupuncture needle, or even a sham needle, since even pricking the skin will involve the inflammatory response, and at the very least an acupuncture treatment involves the modulation of the inflammatory system. The alternative offered is to needle a point or an area on the body that is not related to the condition being treated. But, how is it known that the point or area does not influence the condition being treated?[39] Even pressing the skin? There is evidence that massage modulates endorphin secretion, and so a sham acupuncture technique that involves pressing on the skin will most likely alter the neuroendocrine environment, whether the sham is pressing the same points used in the point prescription being assayed, or is a different point prescription entirely.

In terms of manual acupuncture, it seems to me that until a specific treatment is shown to reliably cause a specific change in biochemicals, a placebo for manual acupuncture is nigh impossible. However, such a possibility for a reliable and consistent approach is beginning to be developed in the use of electro-acupuncture. Electro-acupuncture delivers frequency and amplitude of stimulation that is consistent.

Clinical skills: is the patient narrative necessary in IVF?

Carl Jung once said, 'Learn the theory well, and put it aside when you meet the miracle of another soul.'

From the Program in Placebo Studies & Therapeutic Encounter, we begin to see a group of factors that are thought to be necessary to elicit or even enhance the placebo effect, since the placebo effect is almost certainly mobilised by the time a patient walks into the clinic. The elicitation of the placebo effect appears to rely on empathy, duration of interaction and positive attitude. Recently, developments point to the placebo as many faceted, that there is not one placebo effect but many, each activating a different mechanism, and that a placebo is the 'entire ritual of the therapeutic act'.[40] To elicit such a powerful effect would require a different therapeutic act for each mechanism required and puts much more emphasis on doctor–patient interaction and the patient narrative.

There are conflicting reports over what exactly empathy is, the use of empathy in the clinical setting, and whether it's a good idea to use it at all. Some suggest that being able to learn empathy may not be possible, or the use of empathy in the therapeutic environment may hinder therapy, or that it may not be possible to provide empathy in the clinic in any case.[41] Often, ethics forms part of the argument against the use of empathy in a clinical environment, that the use of empathy may interfere with the objectivity a physician requires in deciding a treatment strategy; 'and the least of these is empathy' pretty much sums up this view.[42] Even if such objectivity were possible, it's difficult to imagine (or even empathise with) what kind of world view would be necessary to be able to present such objectivity.

In contradistinction, the perspective offered by P.D. Maclean, one of the leading brain scientists of the twentieth century, presents entirely the opposite view:

> Above all, medicine is a profession devoted to caring for other individuals... It depends first of all on empathy, the capacity to identify one's own feelings and needs with those of another person... It is the ability to 'look inward' for obtaining insight required for foresight in promoting the welfare of others.[43]

Although the potential of the placebo effect can significantly improve the health of a patient in some conditions, its effect is variable. The variation depends on the patient receiving the medicine, either allopathic or medical technique. However, practitioner technique is essential. Over 50 years ago an editorial in the *BMJ* reported that:

> it is a fallacy to suppose that an inactive medicine can do no harm. If prescribed in a perfunctory way for a patient needing explanation and reassurance it may increase faith in his disease rather than in the remedy, and a doctor who gives a placebo in the wrong spirit may harm the patient.[44]

The disease state is an expression of a somatic dis-ease. The conscious intent of the patient in seeking healing is a reflection of somatic guidance, the unconscious. It could be argued (and is, in psychoanalytic circles) that the patient is consciously seeking relief from the somatic dis-ease, and at the same time at an unconscious level is seeking an awakening of their own slumbering internal healer. Since the placebo effect seems to rely, at least in part, on the physician's ability to elicit it, it is down to the physician to help the patient mobilise their own internal resources as much as possible.

That an acupuncture treatment is not simply the mechanical application of needle insertion is a guiding principle, established in the classics and still guiding practitioners today. In an article published in 1990, Larre and Rochat de la Vallee point out that 'The most important thing for healing is the relationship of the practitioner, the spirits and the patient.'[45]

It could be argued that the modern practice of acupuncture in China might be more mechanical than that practised in the West, but this would be a superficial assessment. Attitudes and practices to health and healing are cultural. The practice of acupuncture in the West appears to be different to its practice in the East, and this is probably a reflection of cultural attitudes to healing and illness.

Acupuncture practised in the East is invariably ward based, and consultations are not necessarily private. I have read accounts of initial consultations in hospitals in China where the consulting room is open; other patients stand by the door listening to the consultation and offering advice to both patient and doctor. Bearing in mind that both social isolation and ill health induce the stress response, and that ill health leads very quickly to social isolation, a healing environment that is socially inclusive could be very beneficial for patients. An example of this in the West is the survival rate of those patients participating in breast cancer support groups, although some questions still remain. The initial trial from 1989 found a significant difference between survival rates in the women participating in it; women in breast cancer support groups survived longer than those who didn't. However, the trial was criticised for using an average rather than median score.[46]

In his later 2007 trial, Spiegel found no difference between two groups of patients suffering from metastatic cancer. However, the trial did identify a significant difference within a sub-group of patients suffering from an aggressive form of cancer, a very interesting finding.[47]

Depression is a known marker of mortality in cancer patients[48] and major depression may be a predictive factor for breast cancer,[49] it is thought by diminishing the strength of the immune system. In elderly people it has been found that chronic depression significantly increases the risk of contracting cancer,[50] whereas elderly patients who are happy and have good emotional health are more likely to survive cancer.[51]

Acupuncture does involve the modulation of the inflammatory response, and neuroendocrines. Hormones, neurohormones and the inflammatory response affect the way that we feel, our internal and external dialogues.

Empathy, the ability to understand and identify at a feeling level the distress another person is experiencing, is an ancient concept. Now, technological developments have begun to illustrate some of the physiological pathways by which people can 'feel' the discomfort of the patient, in some way.[52, 53] This has immediate implications for clinical practice. First, it brings to light and makes us more aware and conscious of our own empathy, and second, because both placebo effect and its other side, nocebo effect, can be elicited in a patient by the physician's own demeanour.

Nevertheless, if the medical practitioner can 'feel' or even appreciate at some level what is going on in a patient, then it's most likely that, in spite of the distress a patient will be experiencing, at some level the patient will be able to feel what is going on in the medical practitioner. In addition to the skills and abilities that may be involved in mobilising the placebo effect, then, congruency is also necessary. Congruency does not necessarily require rapport-building skills, but it will certainly help.

10

Acupuncture in ART

The purpose of this chapter is to go over some details of acupuncture treatments as adjuncts to assisted reproduction technologies that have been shown to improve patient experience and patient response to technological treatments for sub-fertility. Apart from stress, this chapter does not review acupuncture treatments for primary or secondary sub-fertility conditions, such as polycystic ovarian syndrome or endometriosis. There are plenty of very good books on the shelf that provide guidance for those conditions. When we are dealing with patients who have received a diagnosis of sub-fertility, then they are either going to receive a Western conventional remedy for a period of time, such as clomid, or they are going to begin an IVF cycle in the near future or have already begun a cycle, so it is to support that endeavour that our skills must be focused.

Stress in IVF

The concept of stress in the West is stratified according to biochemical assay, the relationship between motivation and workload, and physiological and psychological pathogenesis. It would be easy to say that the general understanding of stress is that at any given time, a person has more to deal with than they can comfortably manage. On the one hand this is reasonable. On the other, comfort is relative and stress is endemic. In some ways we live in much more interesting times than our predecessors, and from the data, our lives are much more stressful.

Stress is truly endemic. In the fertility world, stress is thought to be one of the major causes of sub-fertility. Thereafter, diagnosis of sub-fertility creates stress, the treatment of sub-fertility creates stress, and failed IVF cycles create stress. Many think that fertility treatment should begin by treating stress.

It's necessary to develop a meaningful concept, not only because stress is so prevalent in our society, and not just because it is suggested that the IVF cycle should begin with treatment of stress, but also because the majority I have treated have begun their consultation either by stating directly that they are feeling 'stressed out', or using terms that can quite easily be translated as stress, for example, saying that they feel a total lack of control over the process, or expressing feelings of isolation.

A review published by the *Human Reproduction Update*[1] evaluated 706 articles published over 25 years that related to emotional aspects of IVF treatment. The authors found that in comparison to women who were only just starting their IVF treatment, women that had already experienced one failed cycle appeared to adjust well. However, a 'considerable' group expressed sub-clinical emotional problems as well.

Patients who are in treatment cycles are suffering from stress. Unsurprisingly, over the years papers have been repeatedly published showing that stress, concomitant with IVF treatment, has been the cause of treatment discontinuation, a great sadness for people suffering from sub-fertility and wanting to start a family.

A cohort study published in 2009 found that about 50 per cent of couples drop out before any fertility treatment starts, and about 30 per cent drop out after the first IVF cycle. The main reasons cited in this article were emotional stress and poor prognosis.[2] Around the same time, a questionnaire study received responses from 732 couples, about 55 per cent of the total questionnaires sent. Of these, 515 had discontinued treatment; around 50 per cent (266 people) discontinued treatment because they had achieved a live birth. Of those who had not achieved a live birth, a proportion discontinued treatment because of lack of funding (23%), lack of success (23%) and psychological stress (36%, almost ninety of the remaining 249 not achieving live birth). The authors conclude that better information and support are required.[3]

This finding, that psychological stress is the main reason for ending treatment (excluding live birth), is reflected in a retrospective study published in 2009, where the psychological burden of the IVF cycle was also the main reason for treatment discontinuing.[4]

Reducing the psychological stress might be achievable by incorporating such a service in the IVF treatment strategy, something worth considering when discussing treatment options. Drop-out rates appear to be reduced by changing the type of IVF cycle, that is, by choosing mild IVF (mild ovarian hyperstimulation) along with single embryo transfer. In one study the association between baseline anxiety and drop-out rate was reduced by more than 50 per cent when patients chose mild IVF. [5]

On their website, the American Society for Reproductive Medicine (ASRM) acknowledges that IVF stressors are multifaceted and provides advice on some of the challenges a couple might expect when starting down the IVF route.[6] As long ago as 1987, patients reported a feeling of loss of control as a result of IVF treatment.[7] The number reported at that time was 77 per cent.

Treatment of IVF patients with acupuncture

There is a difference between acupuncture for egg collection and embryo transfer, and acupuncture treatments during pre-egg collection time. The reason for this is that treatment for egg collection and embryo transfer acupuncture are acute, and often use point prescriptions, whereas the time preceding egg collection relates more to chronic conditions and point prescriptions will therefore be unique.

TCM is a very effective system for the treatment of fertility. Its methods and techniques are pragmatic and flexible, originating in antiquity and consistently evolving over centuries, selecting, discarding and developing in a manner very similar to the quality management methods of today; review, action and review. Since those early times the most recent innovation is the integration of TCM with Western conventional medicine. The two systems have much to offer each other.

It may be that patients enter your clinic at the beginning of the fertility journey. Even six months prior to IVF can be beneficial for a patient. Generally however, patients arrive at the clinic after they've started their fertility treatment. So the time available to effect change in their presenting condition(s) is limited by the amount of time prior to egg collection, which may be up to six weeks, and is usually much less. Treatment options are therefore limited. Even within those limitations, however, there is a lot that acupuncture treatments can help with. If the cycle is successful, then that's great!

If the cycle is not successful, then it may be possible to provide treatment that may alleviate problems at a deeper level if a longer lead-in time is made available.

In the event that a patient has only a few weeks prior to egg collection, the main strategies should be to help the patient manage the psychological burden of the IVF cycle, to support the cycle, and to manage any pre-existing conditions that might arise. Often this latter strategy means palliative care.

Insofar as this is the case, then, the key areas to consider supporting are the Sanbao, the Three Treasures (Jing [Essence], Qi [Energy] and Shen [Spirit]), blood flow and stress.

Supporting the cycle

The ancient adage: same disease, different treatment; different disease, same treatment applies in this specialty.

Protocols in IVF (addressed previously) will follow the same pattern with some minor changes. Initially the primary difference will be between the long protocol and other treatment protocols. However, in the event of repeated failed IVF cycles, other treatment strategies will need to be brought to bear, relating to the type of problem being addressed and to support the IVF clinic treatment strategy. A robust strategy to regulate the immune system will be required if the patient is still under the care of the clinic. For example, if intralipids are being used then acupuncture prescriptions should be focused on supporting that treatment; attention to changes in the pulses, which will reflect the nature of the treatment (i.e. slippery), can provide an indication on how things are going. If the result of a failed IVF cycle is down to poor ovarian response, or even ovarian failure, then acupuncture to improve ovarian response and folliculogenesis via blood flow, spleen, kidney and/or heart qi tonification should be the focus. A lot depends on the outcome of the original diagnosis. Often, a suggestion to take a break between treatments, not least to help a patient recover from the previous treatment cycle, can be beneficial. Such a suggestion relies on a patient's needs, however.

The long protocol involves down-regulations plus stimulations. Given that each person is unique and the miracle of another soul, it is not possible to provide a point prescription that will address all the symptoms that a patient may experience as a result of the down-regulations. However, it is possible to think about reasonable strategies.

The down-regulations inhibit ovarian function, so we know that there will be side effects related to both qi stagnation and yin obstruction or depletion, and these usually occur simultaneously. Patients' complaints often reflect the side effects of the pharmaceuticals, which include night sweats, hot flushes, headaches (which can be severe), bloatedness, and feeling tetchy and emotional. Stress as a result of the fertility treatment process will exacerbate many symptoms and so it's important to look out for symptoms of anxiety and depression.

In most cases a protocol that involves the release of liver constraint is a guiding principle, and from that point prescription building out to include *shen* calming points, moving qi associated with whichever elements/organ systems seem most affected by the down-regulation drug and the constraint of qi. The use of a point prescription to alleviate liver constraint is beneficial in a number of ways, not least because every patient will be coping with a large amount of stress, but also because a down-regulation such as buserelin is metabolised by the liver (and kidneys).[8] So supporting these organs is an important safeguard.

In addition to managing the liver constraint, other point prescriptions can be developed to manage the symptoms of yin deficiency and empty heat such as night sweating.

Treatments to manage the side effects of the down-regulations can be provided alongside preparing the patient for ovarian hyperstimulation. In fact, since blood is the mother of qi, and qi is the commander of blood, focusing on moving blood can be an effective treatment to help with constrained energy. There are some good treatments to enhance blood flow to the reproductive system, in addition to the traditional point prescriptions.

Blood flow to the reproductive system

Ovarian response relies on nurture in the form of oxygenated blood and nutrients. Nurture is provided directly by the ovarian arteries. Branches of both the ovarian and the uterine artery unite with each organ, in a form of reproductive arterial anastomosis.

In 1996, the effect of electro-acupuncture on blood flow in the uterine arteries was evaluated. Blood flow was measured in terms of the pulsatility of the uterine arteries, the pulsatility index (PI). This excellent trial not only established an efficacious treatment, but also suggested a potential pathway for the way that it might work; that the application of the differing frequencies, 2Hz and 100Hz, caused changes in different opioid secretion which caused dilation of the uterine arteries. The treatment was supplied twice a week over four weeks.[9]

The trial has been replicated several times, and each replication has found the same effect, that electro-acupuncture of modulating frequencies 2Hz and 100Hz improves blood flow in the uterine arteries. The most recent replication provided by Mo and colleagues (2009) changed the number of treatments from eight treatments over four weeks to four treatments over two weeks, and even with this reduced frequency of treatments found an increase in blood flow in the uterine arteries.[10]

As with the studies, in clinical application I have found that this treatment improves flow of the uterine arteries and improves uterine vascularity, usually demonstrated by a good tri-laminar endometrium on ultrasound and better follicular recruitment. In general, patients also feel better and more relaxed.

Arterial blood flow relies on sympathetic nerve activity, and the vasoconstriction derived from the sympathetic system maintains arterial blood pressure. However, an overactive sympathetic nervous system increases constriction and can impede blood flow.[11] In their write up, Stener-Victorin and colleagues suggested several pathways which might increase blood flow, of which the increased secretion of beta-endorphins derived the 2Hz stimulation is just one.

There are several questions that immediately spring to mind and have yet to be asked of this treatment. Is the uterine environment modulated at all? Is there any change in follicle quantity? Is there any change to follicle quality? In the past these sorts of questions were possible to ask but not possible to explore. Not so with today's technology.

As well as electro-acupuncture, manual acupuncture is often used with well-known points to strengthen the energy of organs known to be involved in blood and the movement of blood. Moxa is often applied, but with an eye to contraindications and the stage of the cycle it can be a difficult adjunct to incorporate.

Egg collection

Egg collection involves sedation and painkillers prior to the usual method of retrieval, using a transvaginal ultrasound. The probe is inserted through the vagina and is used to identify the follicles that have reached maturity. Each follicle is pierced by a thin needle (inserted through an ultrasound guide) and the follicular fluid (which contains the egg) is drawn out using a suction device called an aspirator. The entire operation can take less than an hour and recovery is usually 24 to 48 hours.

Another method of egg collection, which may be used if the ovaries are difficult to reach via transvaginal ultrasound, is a laparoscopy, where a laparoscope, a thin probe, is passed through the abdomen to guide the needle.

SIDE EFFECTS OF EGG COLLECTION

Patients often report some side effects of the egg collection. Usually these are mild and include cramping, abdominal bloating, nausea, dizziness and dull pain. Sometimes there may be spotting and shortness of breath.

Acupuncture treatments for egg collection

In 1999 a Swedish research team published a trial evaluating the use of analgesic acupuncture in comparison to a group who used the anaesthetic alfentanil. Both groups received a paracervical block (PCB). The trial was a success insofar as patient recovery was quick, with less nausea, pain and stress than the anaesthetic group, and although unlooked for and not one of the primary goals, there was an increase in pregnancy rates. The majority of patients stated they would use the method again.[12]

In 2003 the Swedish group published the results of a larger and multi-centre trial. The parameters were the same but for the added evaluation of neuropeptide y (NPY) in follicular fluid and an assessment of pregnancy outcomes. All patients received a PCB; the EA (electro-auricular acupuncture) group received EA and PCB, whereas the control received alfentanil and PCB. The trial found a significantly higher expression of NPY in follicular fluid in the EA group compared with the control, and as with the earlier trial, patient recovery was much quicker and less eventful (in terms of nausea and stress) than in the control. The pregnancy rates between groups were the same.[13]

A similar trial evaluating the effect of electro-auricular acupuncture (EA) as an adjunct to analgesia at egg collection was published in 2006.[14] This trial had three arms: EA, auricular acupuncture (A) and analgesia with remifentanil (CO). The EA group received electro-auricular acupuncture at continuous 1Hz which was self-administered as per patient requirements, the A group received auricular acupuncture to ear points 29, 55 and 57, and the CO group received the application of adhesive tape on the same points as the auricular groups in addition to the analgesia remifentanil.

Again, the results were significant. In comparison to the CO group, the EA group showed a significant increase in wellbeing scores, expressed by both subjective scoring and by the reduced requirement of analgesia. Although the EA group also showed significantly less tiredness than the CO group, all three groups had comparable rates of nausea, most likely due to the use of remifentanil PCB block by all groups. Pregnancy rates in the EA group were also significantly higher than in either the A or CO groups.

Although further trials need to be undertaken, these treatments provide useful adjuncts for patients seeking alternatives to standard care. In addition, they are time saving, cost effective and, as far as the evidence shows, significantly reduce the side effects inherent in the anaesthetics, permitting an earlier recovery and discharge.

The minor surgery for egg collection along with the anaesthetic load, although necessary, is an internal interference of the reproductive system and so it's unsurprising that qi stagnation symptoms occur – the cramping, abdominal bloating and nausea for example. Once again, acupuncture points to move blood and alleviate pain and nausea are the most effective methods for post-egg collection recovery.

Acupuncture for embryo transfer

The first large randomised controlled trial evaluating use of acupuncture for embryo transfer was Paulus *et al.* 2002.[15] This trial investigated the use of two point prescriptions on 80 patients at the time of their embryo transfer (ET); a pre-ET treatment was provided immediately before the ET, and a post-ET treatment was provided immediately after. The control arm consisted of patients who were having ET and did not receive any acupuncture treatments.

The trial was a great success, for patients, for the acupuncture profession and for IVF clinics. The control arm had a 26 per cent clinical pregnancy rate, whilst the intervention arm showed a 42 per cent clinical pregnancy rate.

This initial trial precipitated a rash of further trials, some with different point prescriptions, some with the same point prescriptions, and some trials with different treatment strategies, enough trials for meta-analyses to begin assessing the direction of the data and provide guidance to clinicians on the best advice to provide patients. Early meta-analyses found that overall the provision of acupuncture treatments immediately before and after ET did indeed increase the chances of clinical pregnancy.

Using a point prescription very similar to that used in the Paulus et al. trial of 2002, at an IVF centre we also found that the acupuncture treatments significantly improved clinical pregnancies. In 2009 we published a retrospective analysis of 70 patients who received acupuncture treatments before and after ET compared to 70 controls that were matched for age, day of transfer, and transfer type. As with the Paulus trial, this analysis showed a significant increase in successful clinical pregnancy rates in patients having acupuncture before and after transfer. Interestingly, the effect of the acupuncture treatments increased as age increased: in women younger than 35, 26.3 per cent had a clinical pregnancy in the normal IVF group, whereas in the IVF plus acupuncture group the clinical pregnancy rate was 35 per cent. In the group aged 35 to 39, the clinical pregnancy rate in the normal IVF group was 28.6 per cent whereas the IVF plus acupuncture group saw a clinical pregnancy rate of 39.3 per cent. In women 40 and over, the normal IVF group had a clinical pregnancy rate of 20 per cent, whereas the IVF plus acupuncture group had a clinical pregnancy rate of 35.5 per cent.

Since those early days, further analyses have evaluated the effect of acupuncture treatments at ET and the evidence now provides an inconclusive picture. The lack of a definitive answer raises questions about the nature of the evidence and the guidance provided to professionals. Two trials published in the last decade are good examples of this, one from 2007 and the other from 2009.

The 2007 trial is a curiosity. It has only ever been published in abstract and was a multi-centre trial; the control arm (which received no sham procedures) recorded a clinical pregnancy rate of 69.9 per cent. The intervention arm (the acupuncture arm) recorded 43 per cent. It has to be asked: a clinical pregnancy rate of nearly 70 per cent is an achievement; are these results normal? Was it one centre that had such a large clinical pregnancy rate? Before any judgement can be made, more details are required.

Methodology is also an issue. The authors of the trial stated that the intention was to evaluate the effect of acupuncture treatments for ET off site. Whereas all other trials have been conducted in an IVF centre, in contrast, this trial required patients in the intervention arm to travel between sites – that is, patients had to travel from home to the acupuncture centre for the pre-ET treatment, then to the IVF centre for ET, then back to the acupuncture centre for the post-ET treatment, then home.[16] Patients in the control group, however, were able to go from home to the IVF centre to home again. Bearing in mind that the day of ET is probably one of the most significant days in a woman's fertility journey, it is quite easy to imagine the stress involved. So, the trial methodology in the 2007 trial is significantly different from other trials.

In 2009, researchers from Hong Kong evaluated ET acupuncture against a sham acupuncture control. In both intervention and control arms the researchers used the same point prescription as Paulus *et al.* (2002), but omitted the auricular acupuncture.

A sham acupuncture technique presupposes that acupuncture treatments work and that the sham doesn't. The sham technique used a needle, which on application, pricked the skin of the recipient, making the recipient think they were part of the intervention arm. In this trial, the practitioner tapped the needle and pricked the skin on the same points being used in the intervention arm. This trial found that the sham 'control' achieved better results than the acupuncture intervention arm! The authors concluded that sham acupuncture 'may not be inert'.[17]

Both these trials provide confounding results and demonstrate the difficulty in developing a good evidence base for acupuncture. In fact, beginning with Paulus (2003), in the last decade sham controlled trials have been used more often than not in the evaluation of the effect of acupuncture treatments in ART, and overall the results seem to demonstrate that sham acupuncture is not inert at all.[18] This confounds the development of potentially useful guidance for clinicians and patients. On the other hand, if sham acupuncture is not inert, then perhaps we are looking at the development of another type of acupuncture technique.

Stress and acupuncture treatments

In addition to sub-fertility and fertility treatment, the causes of stress include financial concerns, social isolation and lack of control. The symptoms of acute and chronic stress are manifold.

The pathogenesis of depression and anxiety is thought to be stress, both acute and chronic. Although I have seen IVF patients suffering from depression, almost every patient relates anxiety explicitly during her initial consultation, or the experience of anxiety is shared by implication.

Ways to help manage stress

Acupuncture is a beneficial treatment for women undergoing assisted reproduction treatments. In fact, women find acupuncture treatments an empowering adjuvant, whether or not the treatments result in pregnancy, and I would suggest this self-actualising step is an intuitive response to stress and part of the process of taking back control.[19] It also appears that acupuncture treatments may reduce miscarriage rates in patients undergoing IVF/ICSI and this is probably also due to the effect of acupuncture on stress suffered by fertility patients.[20]

TCM concepts of stress

Stress as a unique, isolated concept is not identified in TCM. However, excluding major diseases, the Western expressions of stress, anxiety and depression are present in the TCM corpus.

The TCM system relies on the premise: from the simple to the complex (and, to paraphrase Shakespeare, simple truth is often mistaken for simplicity). In TCM, the Heart is the organ that makes Blood, and the Spleen is the origin of Blood. Sorrow and shock will deplete Heart energy. When Heart energy becomes impaired so it becomes depleted, leading to anxiety. If the anxiety does not abate, the depletion increases, impairing the Blood-making function, leading to palpitations, choppy pulse and other symptoms.

This is really exacerbated when other systems become compromised. For example, since the Spleen is the origin of Blood, excessive worry, or other factors that can impair its functions such as eating cold and greasy foods, lack of exercise, or lack of sympathy and sympathetic touch, will result in the deficiency of Spleen energy and therefore impair its ability to provide the precursor of Blood to the Heart. Moreover, from the Five Element specialty, the Heart is the Mother of the Spleen. If there is persistent worry (or another pathogenic factor), then the child of the Heart, the Spleen, will become depleted and seek greater nurture from its mother than usual, depleting the Heart qi.

From the Five Element specialty, the Liver is the home of Anger. Anger is an excellent energy when it is in balance, and can be illustrated as the thrust of energy produced by the early growth of a seed, breaking out and pushing up through the ground. All too often this energy seems to be out of balance. When it is out of balance, the Liver becomes constrained and the flow of energy can stagnate.

Constant obstruction of acquiring one's needs is a classic example of this, leading to repeated frustration. If this is repeated over and again, the Liver will stagnate in a downward spiral, and can eventuate in depression. Depression is also often thought to be a result of repressed anger. In fact, both concepts form the basis in the pathogenesis Liver qi stagnation (LQS). In a small case review from 2004, LQS was the common syndrome associated in the treatment of depression.[21] When the Liver gets upset, it attacks its neighbour the Stomach (often causing nausea at menstruation), impairing the Stomach's function of digestion which, concomitantly, will influence the paired organ of the Stomach, the Spleen.

The Liver is the largest organ in the body, and is the main producer of heat, so when its function of maintaining the smooth flow of qi becomes impaired, an increase of Heat will ensue.

Anything that stagnates will cause Heat. The Heat flows up and assaults the Heart, increasing sensations of anxiety. Heat will congeal fluids causing Phlegm which will be caught and carried in the upward flow of Heat to the Heart, and there begin to obstruct the Orifices of the Heart, naturally increasing anxiety. The pathogenic influences assaulting the Heart will also impair the Heart function to nourish the Kidneys and the Spleen.

Pathogenic Heat is essentially a threat to homeostasis. In effect, homeostasis means balance. Homeostasis is homo sapiens' mechanism (and also present in all other mammals) to ensure a balance in life's processes. When balance comes under threat, the system reacts to try to restore it (hence the term reactive homeostasis). The restoration can be the acute activation of the fight–flight response to avoid danger, or by seeking a substance the lack of which the system understands as a threat to balance (e.g. a physiological addiction), or by triggering an oxidative stress response. Whatever the cause of the threat, or whatever the extent, when balance is threatened, the system becomes stressed.

Thermogenesis, the process of heat production, is controlled hypothalamically. Both the thyroid and the sympathetic nervous system regulate thermogenesis hormonally, the former through thyroxine and the latter through the actions of norepinephrine. Times of emotional stress will initially see an increased secretion of both these hormones, and because the basal metabolic rate is controlled by thyroxine and norepinephrine, an increase in the basal metabolic rate (BMR). A rise in body temperature naturally increases the BMR. When the BMR increases, thyroxine secretion is also increased.

Acupuncture in the treatment of depression

Depression is a known result of stress (and may also be a pathogenic factor), is known to be a result of IVF in some cases, and is thought to influence IVF outcome.

Systematic reviews still provide inconclusive guidance on the use of acupuncture treatments to help manage depression.[22, 23, 24] However, individual trials have found that acupuncture treatments to help patients with depression have shown improvements in symptoms of the condition. Both the range and frequency of treatments may depend on the condition that caused the depression. For example, one trial treating depression considers the primary effect may be due to the modulation of norepinephrine. The authors conclude that it may be very beneficial for patients unable to manage the anti-depressant tricylic amitriptyline.[25]

Another trial evaluating the effect of acupuncture in the treatment of depression found significant improvement. This double blind RCT study evaluated the effect of acupuncture on pregnant women. Patients suffering from acute depression received 12 acupuncture treatments over eight weeks. The blinding was achieved by separating the acupuncturist who made the original assessment, diagnosis, treatment strategy, treatment design needle technique and stimulation from the acupuncturist performing the treatments. Unlike the specific protocols used in the trials at embryo transfer, point prescriptions were individually tailored as a result of TCM consultation and diagnosis. As per unit safety measures, acupuncture points identified in TCM texts that are known to be contraindicated during pregnancy were excluded. These include LI 4, Sp 1, Sp 6, GB 21, GB 44, UB 23, UB 32, UB 60, UB 67, Ren 3, 4, 5 and 6, St 36, St 45, and Kd 4.[26] The success rate of this trial was 69 per cent, comparing well with the 40 per cent usually found in placebo-controlled pharmaceutical trials.[27]

Acupuncture in the treatment of anxiety

Chronic and acute anxiety are both results of stress, and stress is negatively correlated with fertility and IVF.

The common treatments for anxiety are psychotherapy and/ or pharmaceutical regimes. The most frequently purchased treatments, however, are pharmacological anxiolytics, the class of drugs that inhibit anxiety, and the most common anxiolytics are benzodiazepines, also known as tranquillisers. These include trade names such as Valium, Ativan or Xanax. They are usually fast acting and effectively alleviate panic attacks or other symptoms of acute anxiety, but their effect is temporary, and they have side effects.

The side effects of benzodiazepines are significant. They are addictive, cause nausea, impair thinking and establish a lack of energy. As a result, patients often drop out of treatment. As a temporary relief, the actual cause of the anxiety is not addressed, and so once administration of the drug has ceased the ultimate cause of the anxiety will still need to be addressed. The other problem with pharmaceuticals is that they are pharmacokinetically dynamic, interacting with other drugs. Even for those patients who stay the course of treatment, which can be at least a year, any resolution to the presenting condition, whether anxiety or depression, is relatively short lived.[28] Seeking alternatives is imperative.

The immune system is fundamentally involved in fertility. In 2007, a trial evaluated the effect of acupuncture in the treatment of emotional systems thought to be involved in the experience of anxiety, and subsequent immunological changes. The immune response was evaluated in a range of different factors including chemotaxis, phagocytosis and NK.

The trial found that a specific point protocol improved chemotaxis (the process of molecular migration through signalling) of the immune cells. The authors, Arranz *et al.*, state that 'acupuncture treatment of anxiety decreases immune cell adherence, facilitating the migration of cells through the endothelial layer towards the infection focus'.[29]

In addition to the regulation of leukocyte migration, the increase of ROS in anxious women was also reduced by the acupuncture protocol. This has clear benefits for IVF patients, since increased ROS are known to eventually establish a state of oxidative stress in immune cells, leading to compromised chemotaxis and membrane fluidity.[30, 31] ROS are implicated in follicular development, embryo development and the uterine environment.

All immune parameters, whether they were impaired and reduced, or elevated and hyperactive, were brought to parameters similar to or equal to those of healthy controls. The regulatory effect began immediately after the first treatment, and was noticeable after

72 hours. A subgroup of patients received a full treatment cycle of the point prescription, ten sessions over a year until complete remission.

The suggested point prescription to treat anxiety through manual acupuncture involves ten treatments on SI 3, HT 3 and 5, PC 6, LI 4 and 11, TH 5, CV 3, 4, 6 and 15, GB 34 and 43, St 36, Sp 6, Lv 2, UB 60, Kd 6 and GV 20.

Law of minor returns

There is only so much that a person can do, can train, can amend their lifestyle, to improve performance. There are human limitations, and in most sports disciplines the limitations are reached. But still athletes are achieving breakthroughs. I think we can draw some lessons from the sports arena.

Professional cyclists train non-stop. They are at their peak, physically, mentally and emotionally. There is very little that can be done to increase performance in a person when they reach this kind of level. But it's possible to improve outcome by making small changes to the environment, the equipment, dietary habits, food intake, and so on.

Making small changes is used in many fields of activity. Making changes that are possible, that are realistic and achievable is the goal. The good thing about making small changes is that they are easy to stick to. Obviously this changes in the event of a dramatic problem, like drug addiction. However, if losing weight and changing diet is the requirement, then incorporating new foods and excluding the ones that are not healthy can be done at a measured pace. The goal is to make changes that last.

It is the small changes that, when taken overall, can make a significant difference to the outcome. For the last decade I have been suggesting small changes to patients, tilting the balance in the favour of health. Bearing in mind that many patients arrive in the clinic with only a few weeks to go to ET, making large dramatic changes will simply increase stress and mitigate against success. The changes need to be specific, easy to manage and related to timescale. If your patient has started treatment with you three months prior to egg collection, then changes can be consecutive and easily introduced into the treatment plan and lifestyle advice. On the other hand, if your patient has started treatment with you on the day of embryo transfer then whatever advice given (and almost always advice is requested) must be very easy to follow and very easy to incorporate into the lifestyle she projects over the two weeks following embryo transfer.

Other stress management techniques

In the previous chapter the beginnings of the mechanism underlying the placebo were outlined. This is really good news, since to be able to augment treatment by including those attributes involved, such as empathy, duration of interaction and positivity, would ideally bring the placebo effect to bear. Even though these factors are taught, at least in part, in the clinical skills section in colleges it is still useful to keep these in the forefront during patient care.

It is also interesting to note that empathy, a skill that is both natural and technical, can be enhanced by meditative techniques such as mindfulness meditation, yoga and qigong. No wonder then that earlier practitioners of acupuncture advised daily qigong practice.

Mindfulness meditation

This excellent system originates from Buddhist meditation techniques. The leader in the field is probably John Kabat-Zinn and the 'mindfulness-based stress reduction programme' (MBSR). There are many research trials and meta-analyses that confirm the beneficial effects of this practice. The effects of learning the techniques influence sub-clinical stress and clinical conditions derived from stress.

Research into MBSR has been undertaken. As is often the case, however, it has been reported that many studies lack a methodological basis that meets evidence-based criteria. Nevertheless, overall, meta-analyses and trials evaluating it report that patients find relief from stress, recover control, recover a sense of self-esteem and wellbeing, and learn stress and emotion management techniques that enhance their lives.[32, 33] There remains some doubt, although this is mostly in the domain of meta-analyses. A review published in 2007 showed that current evidence was equivocal on the effect of MBSR on anxiety and depression.[34] In the same year, another trial evaluating the effect of MBSR on depression showed significant improvement of symptoms of depression in the intervention arm after an eight-week course[35] and more recently, a further review evaluating the evidence of the effect of MBSR on anxiety and depression reported a robust effect.[36]

In addition to the effect on stress and the ease of learning the techniques, mindfulness seems to inculcate long-term benefits. In many cases, treating stress or clinical conditions such as depression relies on patient adherence to the treatment programme as a prerequisite. As mentioned earlier, patient drop-out often leads to programme failure, and even in the event that patients do maintain treatment, consistent remission is often not a foregone conclusion. However, the effect of mindfulness techniques appears to have a longevity, which is based on maintaining practice over a longer period of time. It is therefore a self-empowering technique. In one study I have read, a one- year follow-up after the completion of the mindfulness course, practice maintenance remained consistent and wellbeing remained elevated.[37]

It would be unrealistic to say that mindfulness only influences emotions, since all emotions correlate with brain activity and hormonal, neuroendocrine response. A recent study evaluating the effect of mindfulness meditation on the clinical condition of social anxiety disorder demonstrated alleviation of symptoms, improved self-esteem and other associated criteria. The authors went a step further and evaluated the effects of the process on brain activity through fMRI. Brain structures associated with stress and emotional reactivity became less active, whilst other structures associated with cognition and attention usually impaired by stress reactions showed increased activity, further confirming the theory of stress reactivity and cognition/attention in brain structures, whilst also establishing a foothold in the homeostatic process.[38]

All in all, mindfulness is a good technique for patients entering into the ART treatment programme.

In addition to mindfulness training, exercise is known to reduce stress and help with symptoms of anxiety. Meditation is also included in Eastern exercise regimes such as yoga, tai chi and qigong. Although there is more published research on the effect of mindfulness on stress and anxiety than in the other systems, in addition to anecdotal evidence, some research evidence does exist. Research reports that both yoga and tai chi are beneficial exercises and show an improvement in symptoms of stress and anxiety.[39, 40] Frankly, it would be a surprise if either of these systems had no effect on stress or anxiety, given that both incorporate mindfulness techniques and exercise.

Laughter therapy

A recent innovative therapy is laughter therapy, and although the therapy is comparatively new it is getting results. In a study from Korea, laughter therapy delivered eight times over two weeks and compared to controls significantly improved symptoms of depression, anxiety and stress in patients suffering from breast cancer. The therapy can influence the immune system and natural killer cell activity, and the renin-angiotensin system in patients with type 2 diabetes.[41, 42, 43] Laughter therapy has been evaluated in the fertility world: in a quasi-randomised study, medical clowning was assessed against a control group and showed significantly increased positive pregnancy rates.[44] It would be an interesting trial to observe!

11 A Return to Diet

Nutritional therapy and dietary advice is a whole discipline in the TCM system and it would require another book to begin to expand on nutritional therapy in the treatment of fertility. However, some general principles can be applied.

The Stomach and Spleen are the origin of energy and Blood (and energy is also derived from the air we breathe). So the type of food eaten is really important generally, and especially when it comes to fertility treatment and IVF.

From a TCM point of view, the digestion of food relies on the energy of the Stomach and Spleen. If the Stomach and Spleen energy is strong, then digestion will be effective. Foods that are more difficult to digest will consume more energy and make the Stomach and Spleen tired. The types of foods that tire the Stomach and Spleen include cold foods, raw foods, greasy foods, and complicated and rich foods.

Cold foods and raw foods impair the energy of the Stomach and Spleen. In the case of cold foods, the Stomach tires more quickly because it must expend energy to warm them up. When it comes to raw foods, the structure of raw food is still strong. Cooking breaks down the structure of food. So, in general it is thought better to cook the food, or partially cook it, to increase its digestibility. The same can be said for drinks; drinks should be room temperature or above. Iced drinks are reserved for very special occasions (if at all). Think of the Stomach and Spleen like a baby; easily digested foods will enhance the process of digestion and lead to effective delivery of the nutrients required for energy and Blood. I've yet to meet a baby who enjoys a freezing cold shower first thing in the morning and I haven't met many adults who like iced showers either.

Dietary supplementation

ROS are a natural result of cellular metabolism. They are also important signalling molecules and support homeostasis when in balance. When out of balance, however, they can become toxic. The states that cause imbalance include stress and heat. Keeping ROS in balance can be managed by dietary supplementation of vitamins and the right foods. If there is a systemic cause, such as liver constraint (as a result of stress, sub-fertility or anxiety/depression for instance), it would be best if acupuncture were provided in addition to dietary supplementation.

Vitamins

The term 'vitamin' is derived from the words 'vital amine' and coined by the Polish–American biochemist Caismir Funk in 1912. Mr Funk learned that people who eat brown rice are less likely to develop the nutritional disease beriberi (*beri* is Sinhalise and means 'weak' – its repetition is to emphasise just how weak a person becomes who is suffering from this nutritional deficiency). His attempt to isolate the core compound (thiamine) led to his isolation of niacin (vitamin B3) and his concept of vital amines.

VITAMIN A

Chemical name: All-trans-Retinol (atROH)

Food source: Liver, dairy, saltwater fish (herring, sardines, tuna), cod and cod liver oil, carrots, corn, dark leafy greens, yellow squash, polar bear liver.

RDA: For women (non-lactating), 770mcg.[1] Five servings of fruit and vegetables will provide roughly 50 per cent of the RDA. Vitamins A, D, and E have been found to interact with vitamin K in some circumstances. Please review information on interactions with Vitamin K on page 158.

VITAMIN B6

Chemical name: Pyridoxal phosphate (active component)

Food source: Main dietary sources include fish, particularly salmon and tuna (yellowfin), organ meats, liver (beef), turkey, chicken (breast), starchy vegetables. Other sources include cottage cheese, chickpeas, potatoes, squash, onions, spinach, watermelon, nuts and raisins, bananas.

RDA: For women (non-lactating), by mouth 20mg;[2] maximum dose 100mg prior to clinical consultation; fertility dose 30mg.

VITAMIN BETA-CAROTENE

Chemical name: β-carotene

Food source: Any fruits/vegetables that are yellow or rich orange; mangoes, papaya, yams, carrots, pumpkins, sweet potatoes, spinach and kale (the red colouring effect is masked by chlorophyll in spinach and kale).[3]

RDA: None noted, because it is an inert precursor to vitamin A. Best eaten at night with a meal containing fat.

Contraindications: In general, this is a very benign substance. However, interactions with cholesterol-lowering pharmaceuticals have been noted. High consumption of beta-carotene increases the risk of lung cancer in smokers and former smokers.

Side effects: If too much is eaten, skin turns orange and looks a little like fake tan.

COENZYME Q10

Chemical name: Ubiquinone

Food source: Primary sources: beef (heart, liver, muscle), pork (heart, liver, muscle), chicken (heart), soybean oil, olive oil, grapeseed oil. Other sources: oily fish (sardine, mackerel, salmon and tuna), nuts and seeds (particularly sesame) and vegetables.

RDA: 30–200mg a day, taken at night with a meal containing fat.[4, 5]

VITAMIN C

Chemical name: L-ascorbic acid

Food source: Main dietary sources include citrus fruits (tomatoes, oranges, grapefruits) and vegetables. Other sources include green vegetables, the super food broccoli, potatoes, green peas, kiwi fruits, red and green peppers.

RDA: For women (non-lactating), by mouth, 75mg.[6] Although evidence for the effectiveness of vitamin C to improve fertility is inconclusive, it has been shown to improve luteal phase and increase endometrial thickness and with no compelling data on adverse effects, a daily dose of 2000mg is considered safe.[7, 8, 9, 10]

VITAMIN D

Chemical name: Calciferol (D3, cholecalciferol, D2, ergocalciferol)

Food source: Main dietary sources are fatty fish (salmon, tuna, mackerel), fish oil (cod liver oil). Other sources include beef (liver), cheese, egg yolks, sardines.

RDA: For women (non-lactating), by sun rays on arms and face for 30 minutes per day. If this is not available, do not take more than about 0.025mg per day.[11] If steroids are prescribed, then advice from a qualified professional should be sought. Vitamins A, D, and E have been found to interact with vitamin K in some circumstances. Please review information on interactions with Vitamin K on page 158.

VITAMIN E

Chemical name: Tocopherol

Food source: Vegetable oils such as sunflowers oils, wheat germ and safflower oils have the highest proportion. Other dietary sources include seeds and nuts such as sunflower seeds, almonds and hazlenuts, nut oils, green vegetables and some fruits like avocado pears.

RDA: 15mg per day.

Pharmcokinetics: Tocopherols have the capacity to interact detrimentally with antiplatelet medication and vitamin K clotting factors. The National Institutes of Health cite studies indicating that taking vitamin E with other antioxidants (such as selenium, vitamin C and vitamin K in conjunction with simvastatin (a phamaceutical administered after heart attacks and taken to reduce cholesterol) and niacin can inhibit the increase in high-density lipoprotein.[12, 13, 14] It is also noted that in the treatment of cancer using radio- or chemotherapies, some oncologists have advised against the administration of vitamin E (or any antioxidants, for that matter), because of the potential inhibiting of oxidative damage in cancerous cells.[15, 16] However, this is still contentious.[17]

VITAMIN K

Chemical name: Vitamin K1, phylloquinone (or phytomenadione); vitamin K2, menaquinones

Food source: Phylloquinone (K1): kale, spinach, collards, swiss chard, mustard greens, turnip greens, broccoli, brussel sprouts, cabbage, asparagus. Menaquinones (K2): natto, goose leg, goose liver pate, chicken liver, chicken breast, hard and soft cheeses, egg yolk, butter.

RDA: 80 micrograms per day.

Pharmcokinetics: Vitamin K (VK) is principally involved in blood clotting, although it has many other functions.

There are two forms of VK. VK1 from plant (leafy green plants) is called phylloquinone and has a saturated phytyl side chain. It is also available through oils (e.g. soya and canola). Phylloquinone is not easily available in it's natural state (from leafy greens).

VK2 called menaquinone can be created by some bacteria (e.g. bacteria found in the gut) and have an unsaturated side chain. There is a range of menaquinones. The menaquinone with the same length of side chain as phylloquinone (called menatetranone or MK-4) is produced in Japan as a medicine for humans. In distinction to VK1, VK2 is produced by some cheeses, or natto (Japanese bean curd fermentation). Research has shown that VK2 significantly reduces the prospect of heart disease, so it is a cardiovascular protector,[18] but also in the event of arterial calcification, a diet high in VK1 and VK2 reduces arterial calcification, and increases the natural ability of calcified arteries to distend.[19]

VK interacts with the blood-thinning medication warfarin (brand name Coumadin). If warfarin has been prescribed, advice and guidance should be sought from a Western medical doctor. The National Institute of Health fact sheet[20] provides that sudden variations in consumption of VK can either increase or decrease the effect of warfarin. The amount consumed should remain consistent until such time as a consultation with a Western medical doctor can be arranged.

Other vitamins interact with VK, including vitamins E, A and D. Vitamin E helps to thin the blood and so may potentiate the effect of warfarin. The NIH fact sheet provides that an IU of 800 may be safe, although this has yet to be confirmed.

Large doses of vitamins A and D may increase VK deficiency, and it has been noted that prothombin levels are reduced even further in patients receiving warfarin or other clotting factor drugs when doses (400 IU) of a-tocopherol (vitamin A) are administered.

Populations at risk from VK deficiency include the following:

1. Foetuses (because VK is not easily transported through the placenta) and babies (as stated above, and also because levels of VK are low in human milk).
2. Antibiotics will kill bacteria, some of which make menaquinones, and so people who have been prescribed antibiotics may be at risk of VK deficiency.

   Some antibiotics also interact with warfarin. Further advice should be sought from a Western medical doctor.
3. Older people, and particularly postmenopausal women.

In the UK, a safe intake was set in 1991:

- for adults, 1ug/kg/day
- for children, 10ug/kg/day.

In the US, an adequate intake was defined as:

- for adult women, 90ug/day
- for adult men, 120ug/day
- for infants (0–6 months), 2ug/day
- for children (aged 7–12 years), 2.5ug/day.[21]

Vitamin K is thought to be non-toxic and so an upper limit (beyond common sense and taste) has not been defined. VK is both a cardio protector and a cardiovascular rejuvenator, so it is right to eat a reasonable amount (reasonable should be understood as an amount that is normally used in general) alongside other foods with no specific restrictions other than common sense and the medical considerations outlined above.

There also is no guidance regarding fertility, but it appears safe in reasonably (as defined in the previous paragraph) large amounts.

FOODS HIGH IN VITAMIN K (EQUAL TO OR MORE THAN 200% OF DAILY VALUE)[22]

Food	Serving size	% daily value
Kale, fresh or boiled	½ cup	660
Spinach, fresh or boiled	½ cup	560
Turnip greens, frozen or boiled	½ cup	530
Collards, fresh or boiled	½ cup	520
Swiss chard, fresh or boiled	½ cup	360
Parsley	¼ cup	300
Mustard greens, fresh or boiled	½ cup	260

FOODS MODERATELY HIGH IN VITAMIN K (60–199% OF DAILY VALUE)[23]

Food	Serving size	% daily value
Brussel sprouts, frozen boiled	½ cup	190
Green leaf lettuce, shredded	1 cup	125
Broccoli, raw, chopped	1 cup	70
Romaine lettuce, raw	1 cup	70

Minerals

In general, minerals required for health are trace elements – that is, not much is needed at all to sustain health. Listed below are some minerals that are important and should be present in a balanced diet.

SELENIUM

Chemical name: Se

Food source: Main dietary sources are: Brazil nuts, seafood (particularly tuna) and offal (i.e. liver and other organs). Other dietary sources include cereals, grains, dairy and meat. However, dietary sources are dependent on the soil.

RDA: For women, 55mcg a day, and during pregnancy 60mcg.

ZINC

Chemical name: Zn

Food source: Main dietary source is oysters. Other dietary sources include red meat and poultry. Otherwise, crab, lobster, dairy products and nuts. Some foods inhibit zinc absorption and these include whole grain breads, cereals and plant foods.

RDA: For women (non-lactating): by mouth 8mg;[24] fertility dose 15mg. Zinc toxicity can occur, causing diarrhoea, nausea, stomach cramps and headaches. For zinc toxicity to occur however, the daily consumption must be four times greater than the amount recommended.

IODINE

Chemical name: I

Food source: Main dietary source is seaweed. Other dietary sources include seafood, dairy products and grains.

RDA: Taking elevated amounts of iodine can cause health problems, and a recent trial found that consumption of 200mcg or more during pregnancy caused overactive thyroid,[25] whereas around 100mcg is sufficient for general consumption.[26] However, levels of iodine in foods varies considerably. For example, it is suggested that a cup of low fat plain yoghurt will deliver roughly 75mcg per serving, but this will depend on where the animal was fed.[27]

General diet

'As above, so below' is one of the (many) ancient sayings in TCM. It illustrates TCM thought on the experience of existing on earth, how we relate to the natural world, how the natural world relates to us. As we move through the world, so it moves through us, physically, in the form of food for instance, immunologically in the form of disease and resistance, and energetically in the many ways that energy influences us. The traditional concepts of circadian rhythms are of particular relevance here.

The rhythm in the flow of nutritive qi, smoothly passing from organ to organ, is one of the bases on which TCM dietary therapy rests and applies principles. A steady diet can keep us healthy. It's best to breakfast like a king, lunch like a prince and sup like a pauper. This is because the time when the stomach is strongest is between seven and nine in the morning; and from nine to eleven in the morning, the spleen is strongest. Corresponding times in the evening relate to the times when the stomach and spleen are at their weakest.

Western thought is beginning to concur. The circadian rhythms of cortisol and insulin, where cortisol has begun its ascendance and insulin its decline, can be thought to reflect the traditional understanding. Evidence also points to the relationship between healthy weight and the TCM 24-hour energy clock. In recent years the association between heart disease and skipping breakfast has become more solid. Studies have evaluated total cholesterol in school children skipping breakfast compared to those who ate breakfast and found the former group had significantly higher levels of total cholesterol than those in the latter group (even those who ate sweets or chips for breakfast), were heavier and had a higher BMI, leading to the conclusion that skipping breakfast could lead to obesity and therefore cardiovascular problems. Trials evaluating adults who habitually skip breakfast not only show an increase in obesity but, also a significantly increased chance of a heart attack.[28, 29, 30, 31, 32, 33] In fact, most research seems to indicate that having a balanced diet that includes at least three meals a day enhances and preserves life.

TCM nutritional therapy differentiates between the 'common' diet and the specific diet; there are common rules that apply across the board, and the previous section illustrates how rejection of some of the rules can lead to ill health. It is, however, impossible to delineate a diet for fertility patients in this work, because everyone is different.

In general, a normal diet might contain 40–60 per cent vegetables, 30–40 per cent grains and around 10–20 per cent meat, dairy or nuts. A patient undergoing Western fertility treatment will already have quite enough excitation going on – a busy life which is usually made busier by an IVF treatment cycle, personal demands and emotions, all of which will put pressure on the digestive system. Diet should be relatively unexciting, and bearing in mind that most spices are moving substances and the goal is to stabilise Blood, spicy food should be avoided (unless it's a treat), along with other difficult-to-digest foods. As mentioned earlier, to increase digestibility, cooking or steaming food is much preferred, particularly since 'the stomach has no teeth'.

Recipes that might be of benefit to patients

RECOVERY CONGEE

This simple recipe is easy to create and beneficial for patients recovering from egg collection, from ET or from another operation. It's comforting and often used to support people recovering from ill health. The recipe can easily be amended to suit individual needs.

½ cup sweet rice

½ cup pearl barley

6 red dates (jujube)

60g (2 ounces) of sweet potato

1 litre (2 pints) of water (or to your preference)

1. Cook in a slow cooker overnight.
2. Before serving, steam some green vegetables to go with it.

BLOOD PORRIDGE

- A cup of rolled oats
- 6 dates (jujube or black dates)
- ½ a pear
- Grated fresh ginger (to taste)
- A cup of water, goat's milk or soya milk

Mix all ingredients together in a bowl.

Blood-forming foods

Women need blood-forming foods (blood is the mother of energy), and this is particularly necessary when it comes to fertility treatment. From a TCM point of view, blood-forming foods include carrots, beetroot, meat such as beef and chicken, dark leafy greens and oily fish.

For IVF patients a good chicken soup is a very useful supplement. Below are two recipes. All ingredients should be organic where possible. At the very least the chicken needs to be organic, since the soup will be drawing out essences from the bones.

RITMEYER FAMILY CHICKEN SOUP

- 1 whole chicken
- 12–16 cups of water (or as many as fill the pan)
- 2 onions
- 3 carrots
- 1 parsnip
- 1 turnip/swede
- 3 celery sticks
- 1 bunch of parsley
- 1 bunch of dill
- Chicken stock
- 1 large knob of ginger
- 2 garlic cloves
- Salt and pepper

1. Wash the chicken and put it into a large saucepan. Add vegetables to the pan. Add water and stock cubes. Tie the herbs in a bunch together and add to pan. Season as required.

2. Cover the pan and bring to the boil. Immediately lower the heat and simmer. Skim the scum off the top and discard.
3. Simmer for two hours.
4. Remove the chicken and divide into pieces.
5. Strain the stock and return as much as needed to the pan. Keep it simmering.
6. Return chicken to pan and add ginger, and other ingredients if required. Simmer for another hour.

CHICKEN NOODLE BROTH[34]

Unlike the previous recipe, quantities in this recipe are for general guidance only, although there are some ingredient-specific suggestions in brackets. The author suggests that the key here is to embrace the concept and then experiment with variations. In this way there is the goodness of the whole chicken, combined with a host of beneficial ingredients and flavours that stimulate the senses and digestion, and nourish the blood.

- Whole organic chicken
- 1 chopped onion
- 4 sticks celery
- 2 sticks lemon grass
- 2 teaspoons ginger
- 2 cloves garlic
- Light miso (live if you can find it)
- 2 limes
- 4 heads pak choi
- 4 spring onions
- Thick noodles
- 1 tablespoon soy sauce
- Knob of ginger, sliced
- Handful of sweet basil
- 200g (7 ounces) mushrooms (shiitake are particularly good)

1. Place a whole organic chicken in a large pot and cover with water. Add a roughly chopped onion and some celery. Bring to the boil, skim and then simmer for around an hour.

2. Remove the chicken and leave it to cool whilst straining the stock and return it to the pan. Put half of the stock to one side for the moment.
3. To make the broth, pour the other half of the stock (or however much is needed) into a pan and add two or three crushed lemon grass stalks (use the base of a saucepan or a rolling pin) a large thumb-sized piece of ginger and two cloves of garlic all finely chopped or minced. Add a tablespoon of light miso.
4. Keep the broth simmering whilst stripping the meat off the chicken. Add as much of the meat as needed and reserve the rest for another meal or two.
5. Now add some noodles. It pays to have good quality noodles as they soften nicely in the soup. Also add the ginger.
6. Add some greens like pak choi, chopped spring onions, a good splash of soy sauce and some lime juice. Right at the end add some sweet basil.
7. Break up the chicken carcass. If there is stock left over, add some more water and add a good dash of white wine vinegar to help release the goodness from the bones. Add some more onion and celery and simmer it for another two hours at least. If there is no stock left over, place the carcass in a pan and cover with water and add two roughly chopped onions, several sticks of celery, and a good dash of white wine vinegar, bring to the boil and then let it simmer for two hours.
8. Strain it off and allow it to cool. It will refrigerate well for three days or freeze for longer.

This dish is extremely nourishing; the bones as well as the meat of the animal are used to create a nutritious, enriching sauce, whilst the spices are used to help digest the richness. Shiitake mushrooms are also important as they combine with chicken to nourish the blood. Adding noodles and vegetables and other mushrooms to the stock means that this dish is very satisfying – it's a classic, and extremely nutritious, one-pot meal.

ENDNOTES

Chapter 1

1. Gutchess AH, Hedden T, Ketay S, Aron A and Gabrieli JDE (2010) Neural differences in the processing of semantic relationships across cultures. *Soc Cogn Affect Neurosci 5*, 2–3: 254–263.
2. Larre C and Rochat de la Valee E (2003) *The Secret Treatise of the Spiritual Orchid (Neijing Suwen Chapter 8)*. Monkey Press, p.1.
3. Teichmann J and Evans K (1999) *Philosophy: A Beginner's Guide*. Oxford: Blackwell Publishing, p.1.
4. Grayling A (1998) *Philosophy 1: A Guide through the Subject*. Oxford: University Press, p.1.
5. Maciocia G (1989) *The Foundations of Chinese Medicine*. Edinburgh: Churchill Livingstone, p.35.
6. Energy: Oxford Concise Science Dictionary (1996) (3rd edition). Oxford: Oxford University Press.
7. Massachusetts Institute of Technology (no date) Review C: Work and Kinetic Energy. http://web.mit.edu/8.02t/www/materials/modules/ReviewC.pdf, accessed 29 July 2014.
8. Maciocia G (1989) *The Foundations of Chinese Medicine*. Edinburgh: Churchill Livingstone, pp.38–59.
9. Cummings M (2013) The latest evidence for acupuncture. London: British Medical Acupuncture Society. www.medical-acupuncture.co.uk/LinkClick.aspx?fileticket=I4kGU27HT_g%3D&tabid=130, accessed 29 July 2014.
10. Cho S-H and Hwang E-W (2010) Acupuncture for primary dysmenorrhoea: a systematic review. *BJOG*, doi: 10.1111/j.1471-0528.2010.02489.x.
11. Kim KH, Kang KW, Kim DI, Kim HJ, *et al.* (2010) Effects of acupuncture on hot flashes in perimenopausal and postmenopausal women – a multicenter randomized clinical trial. *Menopause 17*, 2: 228–230.
12. Stener-Victorin E, Wikland M, Waldenstrom U and Lundeberg T (2002) Alternative treatments in reproductive medicine: much ado about nothing. Acupuncture – a method of treatment in reproductive medicine: lack of evidence of an effect does not equal evidence of the lack of an effect. *Hum Reprod 17*, 8: 1942–1946.
13. Anderson B, Haimovici F, Ginsburg E, Schust D and Wayne P (2007) In vitro fertilization and acupuncture: clinical efficacy and mechanistic basis. *Altern Ther Health Med 13*, 3: 38–48.
14. Stener-Victorin E, Waldenstrom U, Andersson SA and Wikland M (1996) Reduction of blood flow impedance in the uterine arteries of infertile women with electro-acupuncture. *Hum Reprod 11*, 6: 1314–1317.
15. Zeisler H, Eppel W, Husslein P, Bernaschek G and Deutinger J. (2001) Influence of acupuncture on Doppler ultrasound in pregnant women. *Ultrasound Obstet Gynecol* 17: 229–232.
16. Sandberg M, Lindberg LG and Gerdle B (2004) Peripheral effects of needle stimulation (acupuncture) on skin and muscle blood flow in fibromyalgia. *Eur J Pain 8*, 2: 163–171.
17. Newberg AB, Lariccia PJ, Lee BY, Farrar JT, Lee L and Alavi A (2005) Cerebral blood flow effects of pain and acupuncture: a preliminary single-photon emission computed tomography imaging study. *J Neuroimaging 15*, 1: 43–49.
18. Ming Ho, Li-Chia Huang, Yin-Yi Chang, Huey-Yi Chen, *et al.* (2009) Electroacupuncture reduces uterine artery blood flow impedance in infertile women. *Taiwanese Journal of Obstetrics and Gynecology 48*, 2: 148–151.
19. Thiering P, Beaurepaire J, Jones M, Saunders D and Tennant C (1993) Mood state as a predictor of treatment outcome after in vitro fertilization/embryo transfer technology. *J Psychosom Res 37*, 5: 481–491.
20. Gallagher SM, Allen JJ, Hitt SK, Schnyer RN and Manber R (2001) Six-month depression relapse rates among women treated with acupuncture. *Complement Ther Med 9*, 4: 216–218.

21. Tsay SL, Cho YC and Chen ML (2004) Acupressure and transcutaneous electrical acupoint stimulation in improving fatigue, sleep quality and depression in hemodialysis patients. *Am J Chin Med 32*, 3: 407–416.
22. Achache H and Revel A (2006) Endometrial receptivity markers, the journey to successful embryo implantation. *Human Reproduction Update 12*, 6: 731–746.
23. Gonzalez RR and Leavis P (2001) Leptin upregulates beta3-integrin expression and interleukin-1beta, upregulates leptin and leptin receptor expression in human endometrial epithelial cell cultures. *Endocrine 16*, 21–28.
24. Simon C, Frances A, Piquette GN, el Danasouri I, *et al.* (1994) Embryonic implantation in mice is blocked by interleukin-1 receptor antagonist. *Endocrinology 134*: 521–528.
25. Simon C, Gimeno MJ, Mercader A, O'Connor JE, *et al.* (1997) Embryonic regulation of integrins beta 3, alpha 4, and alpha 1 in human endometrial epithelial cells in vitro. *J Clin Endocrinol Metab 82*, 2607–2616.
26. Chen J, Huang C, Xiao D, Chen HP and Cheng JS (2003) Expression of interleukin-6 mRNA in ischemic rat brain after electroacupuncture stimulation. *Acupunct Electrother Res 28*, 3–4: 157–166.
27. Houju Fu, Yuanqiao He, Ying Gao, Yicun Man, Wukun Liu, and Hua Hao (2011) Acupuncture on the endometrial morphology, the serum estradiol and progesterone levels, and the expression of endometrial leukaemia-inhibitor factor and osteopontin in rats. *Evidence-Based Complementary and Alternative Medicine*, Article ID: 606514.
28. Juan Gui, Fan Xiong, Wei Yang, Jing Li, Guangying Huang (2012) Effects of Acupuncture on LIF and IL-12 in rats of implantation failure. *American Journal of Reproductive Immunology 67*, 5: 383–390.
29. Tsuchiya, Masahiko Sato, Eisuke F, Inoue, Masayasu, Asada, Akira (2007) Acupuncture enhances generation of nitric oxide and increases local circulation. *Anesthesia & Analgesia 104*, 2: 301–307.
30. Sheng-Xing Ma (2003) Enhanced nitric oxide concentrations and expression of nitric oxide synthase in acupuncture points/meridians. *The Journal of Alternative and Complementary Medicine 9*, 2: 207–215.
31. Cho ZH, Hwang SC, Wong EK, Son YD, *et al.* (2006) Neural substrates, experimental evidences and functional hypothesis of acupuncture mechanisms. *Acta Neurol Scand 113*: 370–377.
32. Yamaguchi N, Takahashi T, Sakuma M, Sugita T, *et al.* (2007) Acupuncture regulates leukocyte subpopulations in human peripheral blood. *Evidence-Based Complementary and Alternative Medicine 4*, 4: 447–453.
33. Mori H, Nishijo K, Kawamura H, and Abo T (2002) Unique immunomodulation by electro-acupuncture in humans possibly via stimulation of the autonomic nervous system. *Neuro Letters 320*, 1–2: 21–24.
34. Zijlstra F, van den Berg-de Lange I, Huygen F and Klein J (2003) Anti-inflammatory actions of acupuncture. *Mediators of Inflammation 12*, 2: 59–69.
35. Wick F, Wick N and Wick MC (2007) Morphological analysis of human acupuncture points through immunohistochemistry. *American Journal of Physical Medicine & Rehabilitation 86*, 1: 7–11.
36. Liu K, Li AH, Wang W and Xie YK (2009) Dense innervation of acupoints and its easier reflex excitatory character in rats. *Zhen Ci Yan Jiu 34*, 1: 36–42.
37. Ma SX (2003) Enhanced nitric oxide concentrations and expression of nitric oxide synthase in acupuncture points/meridians. *Journal of Alternative and Complementary Medicine 9*, 2: 207–215.
38. Chen B, Chen J, Zhao X, Liu Y, Chen J, Guo Y and Guo Y (2013) Advances of studies on correlation of acupoints with calcium. *World Journal of Acupuncture – Moxibustion 23*, 1: 33–39.
39. Yan XH, Zhang XY, Liu CL, Dang RS, Ando M, Sugiyama H, Chen HS and Ding GH (2009) Imaging study on acupuncture points. *J Phys Conf Ser 186*, 1.
40. Chang W, Weissensteiner H, Rausch WD, Chen KY, Wu LS and Lin JH (1998) Comparison of substance P concentration in acupuncture points in different tissues in dogs. *AJCM 26*, 1: 13–18.
41. Kim SK, Park JH, Bae SJ, Kim JH, *et al.* (2005) Effects of electroacupuncture on cold allodynia in a rat model of neuropathic pain: mediation by spinal adrenergic and serotonergic receptors. *Exp Neurol 195*: 430–436.

42. Kim SK, Lee G, Shin M, Han JB, *et al.* (2006) The association of serum leptin with the reduction of food intake and body weight during electroacupuncture in rats. *Pharmacol Biochem Behav 83*: 145–149.
43. Rho Sam-Woong, Choi Gi-Soon, Ko Eun-Jung, Kim Sun-Kwang, *et al.* (2007) Molecular changes in remote tissues induced by electro-acupuncture stimulation at acupoint ST36. *Mol Cells* 25, 2: 178–183.

Chapter 2

1. Mishra GD, Cooper R, Tom SE and Kuh D (2009) Early life circumstances and their impact on menarche and menopause. *Women's Health 5*, 2: 175–190.
2. Sex Information and Education Council of Canada (2013) Early menarche: Trends, risks and possible causes. http://sexualityandu.ca/uploads/files/CTR_EarlyMenarche_FEB2013-ENG.pdf, accessed 29 July 2014.
3. Mishra GD, Cooper R, Tom SE and Kuh D (2009) Early life circumstances and their impact on menarche and menopause. *Women's Health 5*, 2: 175–190.
4. Maclure M, Travis LB, Willett W, MacMahon B (1991) A prospective cohort study of nutrient intake and age at menarche. *Am J Clin Nutr 54*, 4: 649–656.
5. Petridou E, Syrigou E, Toupadaki N, Zavitsanos X, Willett W and Trichopoulos D (1996) Determinants of age at menarche as early life predictors of breast cancer risk. *D Int J Cancer 68*, 2: 193–198.
6. Giles LC, Glonek GFV, Moore VM, Davies MJ and Luszcz MA (2010) Lower age at menarche affects survival in older Australian women: results from the Australian Longitudinal Study of Ageing. *BMC Public Health 10*: 341.
7. Revelli A, Piane LD, Casano S, Molinari E, Massobrio M and Rinaudo P (2009) Follicular fluid content and oocyte quality: from single biochemical markers to metabolomics. *Reproductive Biology and Endocrinology 7*: 40.
8. Adams SM, Gayer N, Terry V and Murphy CR (2001) Manipulation of the follicular phase: uterodomes and pregnancy – is there a correlation? *BMC Pregnancy and Childbirth 1*: 2.
9. Kabir-Salmanj M, Nikzad H, Shiokawa S, Akimoto Y and Iwashita M (2005) Secretory role for human uterodomes (pinopods): secretion of LIF. *Mol Hum Reprod 11*, 8: 553–559.
10. Nikas G, Drakakis P, Loutradis D, Mara-Skoufari C, *et al.* (1995) Uterine pinopodes as markers of the 'nidation window' in cycling women receiving exogenous oestradiol and progesterone. *Human Reproduction 10:* 1208–1213.
11. Quinn CE and Casper RF (2009) Pinopodes: a questionable role in endometrial receptivity. *Hum Reprod Update 15*, 2: 229–236.
12. Aghajanova L, Stavreus-Evers A, Nikas Y, Hovatta O and Landgren B-M (2003) Coexpression of pinopodes and leukemia inhibitory factor, as well as its receptor, in human endometrium. *Fertil Steril 79*: 808–814.
13. Pauling L, Itano HA, Singer SJ and Wells IC (1949) Sickle cell anemia, a molecular disease. *Science 110,* 2865: 543–548.
14. Williams RJ (1998) *Biochemical Individuality* (2nd edition). New York: McGraw-Hill.
15. Garrod AE (1931) *The Inborn Factors in Disease: An Essay.* Oxford: Oxford University Press. Cited in Weatherall DJ (2010) Molecular medicine: the road to the better integration of the medical sciences in the twenty-first century. *Notes Rec R Soc 64* (Suppl. 1): S5–S15.
16. Le Monnier de Gouville AC, Lippton HL, Cavero I, Summer WR and Hyman AL (1989) A new family of endothelium-derived peptides with widespread biological properties. *Life Sci 45*: 1499–1514.
17. Sudik R, Chari S, Pascher E, Sturm G (1996) Human follicular fluid levels of endothelins in relation to oocyte maturity status. *Exp Clin Endocrinol Diabetes 104*: 78–84.
18. Rodbell M (1980) The role of hormone receptors and GTP-regulatory proteins in membrane transduction. *Nature 284*, 5751: 17–22.
19. Soede-Bobok AA and Touw IP (1997) Molecular understanding of hematopoietin/cytokine receptor signalling defects in hematopoietic disorders. *J Mol Med (Berl) 75*, 7: 470-477.
20. Lee JH, Kim TH, Oh SJ, Yoo JY, *et al.* (2013) Signal transducer and activator of transcription-3 (Stat3) plays a critical role in implantation via progesterone receptor in uterus. *FASEB J 27*, 7: 2553–2563.

21. Takeda K, Noguchi K, Shi W, Tanaka T, *et al.* (1997) Targeted disruption of the mouse Stat3 gene leads to early embryonic lethality. *PNAS* 94, 3801–3804.
22. Teng CB, Diao HL, Ma XH, Xu LB and Yang ZM (2004) Differential expression and activation of Stat3 during mouse embryo implantation and decidualization. *Mol Reprod Dev 69*, 1: 1–10.
23. Yang XO, Panopoulos AD, Nurieva R, Chang SH, *et al.* (2007) STAT3 regulates cytokine-mediated generation of inflammatory helper T cells. *J Biol Chem 282*, 13: 9358–9363.
24. Gao Q, Wolfgang MJ, Neschen S, Morino K, *et al.* (2004) Disruption of neural signal transducer and activator of transcription 3 causes obesity, diabetes, infertility, and thermal dysregulation. *Proc Natl Acad Sci USA 101*, 13: 4661–4666.
25. Mesa RA (2010) Ruxolitinib, a selective JAK1 and JAK2 inhibitor for the treatment of myeloproliferative neoplasms and psoriasis. *IDrugs 13*, 6: 394–403.
26. Zerbini CA and Lomonte AB (2012) Tofacitinib for the treatment of rheumatoid arthritis. *Expert Rev Clin Immunol 8*, 4: 319–331.
27. Dominguez F, Yanez-Mo M, Sanchez-Madrid F and Simon C. (2005) Embryonic implantation and leukocyte transendothelial migration: different processes with similar players? *FASEB J 19*: 1056–1060.
28. Narvekar SA, Gupta N, Shetty N, Kottur A, Srinivas M and Rao KA (2010) Does local endometrial injury in the nontransfer cycle improve the IVF-ET outcome in the subsequent cycle in patients with previous unsuccessful IVF? A randomized controlled pilot study. *J Hum Reprod Sci 3*, 1: 15–19.
29. Nancy P, Tagliani E, Tay C-S, Asp P, Levy DE and Erlebacher A (2012) Chemokine gene silencing in decidual stromal cells limits T cell access to the maternal-fetal interface. *Science 336*, 6086: 1317–1321.
30. UniProt (Swiss-Prot Protein Knowledgebase) (2014) Human cell differentiation molecules: CD Nomenclature and list of entries. www.uniprot.org/docs/cdlist, accessed 29 July 2014.
31. Ley K (2003) The role of selectins in inflammation and disease. *Trends Mol Med 9*, 6: 263–268.
32. Genbacev O, Prakobphol A, Foulk R, Krtolica A, Ilic D, Singer M, et al. (2003) Trophoblast L-Selectin-Mediated Adhesion at the Maternal-Fetal Interface. Science 299: 405–408. Cited in Foulk RA (2012) Implantation of the Human Embryo, in Bin Wu (ed.) Advances in Embryo Transfer. www.intechopen.com/books/advances-in-embryo-transfer/implantation-of-the-embryo, accessed 13 May 2014.
33. Borsig L, Wong R, Hynes RO, Varki NM and Varki A (2002) Synergistic effects of L- and P-selectin in facilitating tumor metastasis can involve non-mucin ligands and implicate leukocytes as enhancers of metastasis. *Proc Natl Acad Sci. 99*, 4: 2193–2198.
34. Gonzalez RR, Rueda BR, Ramos MP, Littell RD, Glasser S and Leavis PC (2004) Leptin-induced increase in leukemia inhibitory factor and its receptor by human endometrium is partially mediated by interleukin 1 receptor signalling. *Endocrinology 145*, 3850–3857.
35. Dimitriadis E, White CA, Jones RL and Salamonsen LA (2005) Cytokines, chemokines and growth factors in endometrium related to implantation. *Hum Reprod Update 11*: 613–630.
36. Fazleabas AT, Kim JJ and Strakova Z (2004) Implantation: embryonic signals and the modulation of the uterine environment – a review. *Placenta 25* (Suppl. A): S26–S3.
37. Dimitriadis E, White CA, Jones RL and Salamonsen LA (2005) Cytokines, chemokines and growth factors in endometrium related to implantation. *Hum Reprod Update 11*: 613–630.
38. Ohbayashi N, Ikeda O, Taira N, Yamamoto Y, *et al.* (2007) LIF- and IL-6-induced acetylation of STAT3 at Lys-685 through PI3K/Akt activation. Biol Pharm Bull 30: 1860–1864.
39. van Mourik MS, Macklon NS and Heijnen CJ (2009) Embryonic implantation: cytokines, adhesion molecules, and immune cells in establishing an implantation environment. *Journal of Leukocyte Biology 85*, 1: 4–19.
40. Kimber SJ (2005) Leukemia inhibitory factor in implantation and uterine biology. *Reproduction 130*, 2: 131–145.
41. Haines BP, Voyle RB and Rathjen PD (2000) Intracellular and extracellular leukemia inhibitory factor proteins have different cellular activities that are mediated by distinct protein motifs. *Molecular Biology of the Cell 11*, 1369–1383.
42. Haines BP, Voyle RB and Rathjen PD (2000) Intracellular and extracellular leukemia inhibitory factor proteins have different cellular activities that are mediated by distinct protein motifs. *Molecular Biology of the Cell 11*, 1369–1383.
43. Ohbayashi N, Ikeda O, Taira N, Yamamoto, Y, *et al.* (2007) LIF- and IL-6-induced acetylation of STAT3 at Lys-685 through PI3K/Akt activation. *Biol Pharm Bull 30*: 1860–1864.

44. Laird SM, Tuckerman EM, Dalton CF, Dunphy BC, Li TC and Zhang X (1997) The production of leukaemia inhibitory factor by human endometrium: presence in uterine flutings and production by cells in culture. *Hum Reprod 12*, 3: 569–574.
45. Laird SM, Tuckerman EM, Dalton CF, Dunphy BC, Li TC and Zhang X (1997) The production of leukaemia inhibitory factor by human endometrium: presence in uterine flutings and production by cells in culture. *Hum Reprod 12*, 3: 569–574.
46. Lédée-Bataille N, Laprée-Delage G, Taupin J-L, Dubanchet S, Frydman R and Chaouat G (2002) Concentration of leukaemia inhibitory factor (LIF) in uterine flushing fluid is highly predictive of embryo implantation. *Hum Reprod 17*, 1: 213–218.
47. Keltz MD, Attar E, Buradagunta S, Olive DL, Kliman HJ and Arici A (1996) Modulation of leukemia inhibitory factor gene expression and protein biosynthesis in the human fallopian tube. *AM J Obstet Gynecol 175*: 1611–1619. Cited in Kabir-Salmani M, Nikzad H, Shiokawa S, Akimoto Y and Iwashita M (2005) Secretory role for human uterodomes (pinopods): secretion of LIF. Mol Hum Reprod 11, 8: 553–559.
48. Aghajanova L, Stavreus-Evers A, Nikas Y, Hovatta O and Landgren B-M (2003) Coexpression of pinopodes and leukemia inhibitory factor, as well as its receptor, in human endometrium. *Fertil Steril 79*: 808–814.
49. Fouladi-Nashta AA, Jones CJP, Nijjar N, Mohamet L, Smith A, Chambers I, Kimber SJ (2005) Characterization of the uterine phenotype during the peri-implantation period for LIF-null, MF1 strain mice. *Developmental Biology 281*, 1: 1–21.
50. Lord GM (2006) Leptin as a proinflammatory cytokine. *ContribNephrol 151*: 151–164.
51. Malik NM, Carter ND, Murray JF, Scaramuzzi RJ, Wilson CA and Stock MJ (2001) Leptin requirement for conception, implantation, and gestation in the mouse. *Endocrinology 142*: 5198–5202.
52. Frisch RE and McArthur JW (1974) Menstrual cycles: fatness as a determinant of minimum weight for height necessary for their maintenance or onset. *Science 185*: 949–951.
53. Judd SJ (1998) Disturbance of the reproductive axis induced by negative energy balance. *Reprod Fertil Dev 10*: 65–72.
54. Crosignani PG, Vegetti W, Colombo M and Ragni G (2002) Resumption of fertility with diet in overweight women. *Reproductive Biomedicine Online 5*: 60–64.
55. Gao Q and Horvath TL (2008) Cross-talk between estrogen and leptin signaling in the hypothalamus. *Am J Physiol Endocrinol Metab 294*, 5: E817–E826.
56. Santollo J, Marshall A and Daniels D (2013) Activation of membrane-associated estrogen receptors decreases food and water intake in ovariectomized rats. *Endocrinology 154*, 1: 320–329.
57. Butera PC and Czaja JA (1984) Intracranial estradiol in ovariectomized guinea pigs: effects on ingestive behaviors and body weight. *Brain Res 322*: 41–48.
58. Ainslie DA, Morris MJ, Wittert G, Turnbull H, Proietto J and Thorburn AW (2001) Estrogen deficiency causes central leptin insensitivity and increased hypothalamic neuropeptide Y. *Int J Obes Relat Metab Disord 25*: 1680–1688.
59. Malik NM, Carter ND, Murray JF, Scaramuzzi RJ, Wilson CA and Stock MJ (2001) Leptin requirement for conception, implantation, and gestation in the mouse. *Endocrinology 142*: 5198–5202.

Chapter 3

1. UN Department of Economic and Social Affairs (2012) World population projected to reach 9.6 billion by 2050 with most growth in developing regions, especially Africa – says UN. *World Population Prospects: The 2012 Revision.* http://esa.un.org/wpp/documentation/pdf/wpp2012_press_release.pdf, accessed 29 July 2014.
2. Boivin J, Bunting L, Collins JA and Nygren KG (2007) International estimates of infertility prevalence and treatment-seeking: potential need and demand for infertility medical care. *Hum Reprod 22*, 6: 1506–1512.
3. Ferraretti AP, Goossens V, de Mouzon J, Bhattacharya S, Castilla JA, Korsak V, Kupka M, Nygren KG and Nyboe Andersen A (2012) Assisted reproductive technology in Europe, 2008: results generated from European registers by ESHRE. *Hum Reprod 27*, 9: 2571–2584.
4. Human Fertilisation and Embryology Authority (2011) Fertility treatment in 2011: trends and figures. www.hfea.gov.uk/docs/HFEA_Fertility_Trends_and_Figures_2011_-_Annual_Register_Report.pdf, accessed 29 July 2014.

5. Azziz R, Woods KS, Reyna R, Key TJ, Knochenhauer ES and Yildiz BO (2004) The prevalence and features of the polycystic ovary syndrome in an unselected population. *J. Clin Endocrinol Metab 89*, 6: 2745–2749.
6. Rolland M, Le Moal J, Wagner V, Royère D and De Mouzon J (2013) Decline in semen concentration and morphology in a sample of 26,609 men close to general population between 1989 and 2005 in France. *Human Reproduction 28*, 2: 462–470.
7. Irvine S, Cawood E, Richardson D, MacDonald E and Aitken J (1996) Evidence of deteriorating semen quality in the United Kingdom: birth cohort study in 577 men in Scotland over 11 years. *BMJ 312*, 7029: 467–471.
8. Jarvi K, Lo K, Fischer A, Grantmyre J, *et al.* (2010) CUA guideline: the workup of azoospermic males. *Canadian Urological Association Journal 4*, 3: 163–167.
9. National Institute for Clinical Excellence (2013) Guideline 156: Fertility. www.nice.org.uk/guidance/cg156/resources/cg156-fertility-costing-report2, accessed 29 July 2014.
10. Human Fertilisation and Embryology Authority (2009) Intrauterine insemination (IUI) – chance of success. www.hfea.gov.uk/iui-success-rate.html, accessed 15 June 2014.
11. Oxford University Press (2005) The early days of IVF outside the UK. *Hum Reprod Update 11*, 5: 439–460.
12. Human Fertilisation and Embryology Authority (2012) Long-term data treatments. www.hfea.gov.uk/2586.html, accessed 15 June 2014.
13. Human Fertilisation and Embryology Authority (2010) Fertility facts and figures 2008. www.hfea.gov.uk/docs/2010-12-08_Fertility_Facts_and_Figures_2008_Publication_PDF.PDF, accessed 15 June 2014.
14. Human Fertilisation and Embryology Authority (2011) Fertility treatment in 2011: trends and figures. www.hfea.gov.uk/docs/HFEA_Fertility_Trends_and_Figures_2011_-_Annual_Register_Report.pdf, accessed 15 June 2014.
15. Wang J and Sauer MV (2006) In vitro fertilization (IVF): a review of 3 decades of clinical innovation and technological advancement. *Ther Clin Risk Manag 2*, 4: 355–364.
16. Human Fertilisation and Embryology Authority (2011) Fertility treatment in 2011: trends and figures. www.hfea.gov.uk/docs/HFEA_Fertility_Trends_and_Figures_2011_-_Annual_Register_Report.pdf, accessed 29 July 2014.
17. *Mail Online* (2012) Number of IVF babies passes 5m worldwide with demand for techniques still rising. www.dailymail.co.uk/health/article-2167509/Number-IVF-babies-passes-5m-worldwide-demand-techniques-rising.html, accessed 15 June 2014.
18. *Indian Express* (2010) Thirty million couples in India suffer from infertility (10 March). http://archive.indianexpress.com/news/-30-million-couples-in-india-suffer-from-infertility-/588934, accessed 13 May 2014.
19. NHS Choices (2013) IVF: Introduction. www.nhs.uk/conditions/IVF/Pages/Introduction.aspx, accessed 29 July 2014.
20. Human Fertilisation and Embryology Authority (2012) Private fertility treatment. www.hfea.gov.uk/fertility-treatment-cost-private-clinic.html, accessed 29 July 2014.
21. Klerx E (2013) IVF for 200 euro per cycle. www.eshre.eu/Londen2013/Media/Releases/Elke-Klerckx.aspx (2013) accessed 31 July, 2013.
22. Klerkx EPF, Janssen M, van Blerkom J, Campo R and Ombelet W. First pregnancies with a simplified IVF procedure: a crucial step to universal and accessible infertility care. Cited in *Hum Reprod 28*: i4–i6. http://humrep.oxfordjournals.org, accessed 13 May 2014.
23. United Nations Children's Fund and World Health Organisation (2004) *Low Birthweight; Country Regional and Global Estimates.* New York: UNICEF.
24. Goldenberg RL and Culhane JF (2007) Low birth weight in the United States. *Am J Clin Nutr 85*, 2, 5845–5905.
25. Fauque P, Jouannet P, Davy C, Guibert J, *et al.* (2009) Cumulative results including obstetrical and neonatal outcome of fresh and frozen-thawed cycles in elective single versus double fresh embryo transfers. *Fertil Steril 94*, 3: 927–935.
26. Gelbaya TA, Tsoumpou I and Nardo LG (2009) The likelihood of live birth and multiple birth after single versus double embryo transfer at the cleavage stage: a systematic review and meta-analysis. *Fertil Steril 94*, 3: 936–945.
27. Kyrou D, Kolibianakis EM, Fatemi HM, Tarlatzi TB, Devroey P and Tarlatzis BC (2011) Increased live birth rates with GnRH agonist addition for luteal support in ICSI/IVF cycles: a systematic review and meta-analysis. *Human Reproduction Update 17*, 6: 734–740.

28. Davies MJ, Moore VM, Willson KJ, Van Essen P, Priest K, Scott H, Haan EA and Chan A (2012) Reproductive technologies and the risk of birth defects. *N Engl J Med 366*:1803–1813.
29. Martins WP, Rocha IA, Ferriani RA and Nastri CO (2011) Assisted hatching of human embryos: a systematic review and meta-analysis of randomized controlled trials. *Human Reproduction Update 17*, 4: 438–453.
30. Human Fertilisation and Embryology Authority (2009) Assisted hatching. www.hfea.gov.uk/assisted-hatching.html, accessed 31 July 2013.

Chapter 4

1. Dominguez F, Gadea B, Mercader A, Esteban FJ, Pellicer A and Simón C (2008) Embryologic outcome and secretome profile of implanted blastocysts obtained after coculture in human endometrial epithelial cells versus the sequential system. *Fertil Steril 93*, 3: 774–782.
2. Barmat LI, Liu H-C, Spandorfer SD, Xu K, Veeck L, Damario MA and Rosenwaks Z (1998) Human preembryo development on autologous endometrial coculture versus conventional medium. *Fertil Steril 70*, 6: 1109–1113.
3. Peippo J, Viitala S, Virta J, Raty M, *et al.* (2007) Birth of correctly genotyped calves after multiplex marker detection from bovine embryo microblade biopsies. *Molecular Reproduction and Development 74*: 1373–1378.
4. Ipate I, Bogdan AT, Toba LG, Toba GF and Ivana S (2007) Research regarding the embryo biopsy for sexing and genetic testing the bovines embryos. *Revista Romana de Medicina Veterinara 17*: 213–218.
5. Lopatarova M, Cech S, Krontorad P, Holy L, Hlavicova J and Dolezel R (2008) Sex determination in bisected bovine embryos and conception rate after the transfer of female demi-embryos. *Veterinarni Medicina 53*, 11: 595–603.
6. *New York Times* (1993) Scientist clones human embryos, and creates an ethical challenge. www.nytimes.com/1993/10/24/us/scientist-clones-human-embryos-and-creates-an-ethical-challenge.html, accessed 18 May 2014.
7. National Human Genome Research Institute (2014) Cloning. www.genome.gov/25020028, accessed 18 May 2014.
8. US Food and Drug Administration (2010) Animal cloning. www.fda.gov/AnimalVeterinary/SafetyHealth/AnimalCloning/default.htm, accessed 31 July 2013.
9. National Advisory Board on Ethics in Reproduction (1994) Report on human cloning through embryo splitting: an amber light. *Kennedy Institute of Ethics Journal 4*, 3: 251–281.
10. Rosenberg L, Palmer JR, Zauber AG (1994) A case control study of oral contraceptive use and invasive epithelial ovarian cancer. Am J Epidemiol 139: 654–661. Cited in Mahdavi A, Pejovic T, Nezhat F (2006) Induction of ovulation and ovarian cancer: a critical review of the literature. *Fertility and Sterility 85*, 4.
11. Conova S (2003) Estrogen's Role in Cancer: Researchers find oxygen radicals needed for carcinogenesis. In *Vivo 2*, 10. Available at www.cumc.columbia.edu/publications/in-vivo/Vol2_Iss10_may26_03, accessed 25 July 2014.
12. Bhat HK, Calaf G, Hei TK, Loya T and Vadgama JV (2003) Critical role of oxidative stress in estrogen-induced carcinogenesis. *PNAS 100*, 7: 3913–3918.
13. Bouayed J, Rammal H and Soulimani R (2009) Oxidative stress and anxiety: relationship and cellular pathways. *Oxid Med Cell Longev 2*, 2: 63–67.
14. Djuric Z, Bird CE, Furumoto-Dawson A, Rauscher GH, *et al.* (2008) Biomarkers of psychological stress in health disparities research. *The Open Biomarkers Journal* 1: 7–19.
15. Rosenberg L, Palmer JR, Zauber AG (1994) A case control study of oral contraceptive use and invasive epithelial ovarian cancer. Am J Epidemiol 139: 654–661. Cited in Mahdavi A, Pejovic T, Nezhat F (eds) (2006) Induction of ovulation and ovarian cancer: a critical review of the literature. *Fertility and Sterility 85*, 4.
16. Pappo I, Lerner-Geva L, Halevy A, Olmer L, *et al.* (2008) The possible association between IVF and breast cancer incidence. *Ann Surg Oncol 15*, 4: 1048–1055.
17. Salhab M, Al Sarakbi W and Mokbel K. (2005) In vitro fertilization and breast cancer risk: a review. *Int J Fertil Womens Med 50*, 6: 259–266.
18. Arbor L, Narod S, Glendon G, Pollack M, *et al.* (1994) In-vitro fertilization and family history of breast cancer. *Lancet 344*: 611.

19. Ron E, Lunenfeld B, Menczer J, Blumstein T, *et al.* (1987) Cancer incidence in a cohort of infertile women. *Am J Epidemiol 125*, 5: 780–790.
20. Whittemore AS, Harris R and Itnyre J (1992) Characteristics relating to ovarian cancer risk: collaborative analysis of 12 US case-control studies. IV. The pathogenesis of epithelial ovarian cancer. Collaborative Ovarian Cancer Group. *Am J Epidemiol 136*, 10: 1212–1220.
21. Rossing MA, Baling JR, Weiss NS, Moore DE and Self SG (1994) Ovarian tumors in a cohort of infertile women. *N Eng J Med 331*: 771–776.
22. Venn A, Watson L, Bruinsma F, Giles G, Healy D (1999) Risk of cancer after use of fertility drugs with in-vitro fertilization. *Lancet 354*, 9190: 1586–1590.
23. Ness RB, Cramer DW, Goodman MT, et al. (2002) Infertility, fertility drugs, and ovarian cancer: a foiled analysis of case-controlled studies. *Am J Epidemiol 155*: 217–224.
24. van Leeuwen FE, Klip H, Mooij TM, van de Swaluw AM *et al.* (2011) Risk of borderline and invasive ovarian tumours after ovarian stimulation for in vitro fertilization in a large Dutch cohort. *Human Reproduction 26*, 12: 3456–3465.
25. Brinton LA, Trabert B, Shalev V, Lunenfeld E, Sella T and Chodick G (2013) In vitro fertilization and risk of breast and gynecologic cancers: a retrospective cohort study within the Israeli Maccabi Healthcare Services. *Fertility and Sterility 99*, 5: 1189–1196.
26. Hansen M, Kurinczuk JJ, Bower C and Webb S (2002) The risk of major birth defects after intracytoplasmic sperm injection and in vitro fertilization. *N Engl J Med 346*: 725–730.
27. Zhu JL, Basso O, Obel C, Bille C and Olsen J (2006) Infertility, infertility treatment, and congenital malformations: Danish national birth cohort. *BMJ 333*, 7570: 679.
28. Gugucheva M (2010) Malformations in IVF births are a 'public health issue' according to French scientists. www.councilforresponsiblegenetics.org/blog/post/Malformations-in-IVF-Births-are-a-e2809cPublic-Health-Issuee2809d-According-to-French-Scientists.aspx, accessed 1 August 2013.
29. Valbuena D, Jasper M, Remohi J, Pellicer A, Simon C (1999) Ovarian stimulation and endometrial receptivity *Hum Reprod 14* (suppl. 2): 107–111.
30. Pelinck M-J, Keizer MH, Hoek A, Simons AHM, Schelling K, Middelburg K, Heineman MJ (2010) Perinatal outcome in singletons after modified natural cycle IVF and standard IVF with ovarian stimulation. *European Journal of Obstetrics & Gynecology and Reproductive Biology 148*, 1: 56–61.

Chapter 5

1. NHS Choices (2014) Infertility: Introduction. www.nhs.uk/conditions/Infertility/Pages/Introduction.aspx, accessed 29 July 2014.
2. NHS Choices (2012) Trying to get pregnant. www.nhs.uk/Livewell/Fertility/Pages/Getpregnant.aspx, accessed 4 August 2014.
3. World Health Organization (2006) Global database on body mass index. http://apps.who.int/bmi, accessed on 6 October 2013.
4. Weight-control Information Network (WIN) (2010) Prevalence of Overweight and Obesity. http://win.niddk.nih.gov/statistics/#b, accessed 6 Oct 2013.
5. Department of Health (2013) Policy: Reducing obesity and improving diet. www.gov.uk/government/policies/reducing-obesity-and-improving-diet, accessed 29 July 2014.
6. The Poverty Site (2011) United Kingdom: Obesity. www.poverty.org.uk/63/index.shtml, accessed 30 July 2014.
7. Eastwood P, Health and Social Care Information Centre (2014) Statistics on Obesity, Physical Activity and Diet: England 2014. www.hscic.gov.uk/catalogue/PUB13648/Obes-phys-acti-diet-eng-2014-rep.pdf, accessed 30 July 2014.
8. Government Office for Science (2007) Tackling obesities: Future Choices – Project Report (2nd edition). /www.gov.uk/government/uploads/system/uploads/attachment_data/file/287937/07-1184x-tackling-obesities-future-choices-report.pdf, accessed 30 July 2014.
9. Noble RE (2001) Waist-to-hip ratio versus BMI as predictors of cardiac risk in obese adult women. *West J Med 174*, 4: 240–241.
10. World Health Organization STEPwise approach to surveillance (STEPS). www.who.int/chp/steps/en, accessed on 5 June 2014.

11. Zaadstra, BM, Seidell JC, Van Noord PAH, te Velde ER, *et al.* (1993) Fat and female fecundity: prospective study of effect of body fat distribution on conception rates. *BMJ 306*, 6876: 484–487.
12. Shaw JLV, Oliver E, Lee K-F, Entrican G, Jabbour HN, Critchley HOD and Horne Cotinine AW (2010) Exposure increases fallopian tube PROKR1 expression via nicotinic AChRα-7: a potential mechanism explaining the link between smoking and tubal ectopic pregnancy. Am J Pathol 177, 5: 2509–2515.
13. Horne AW, Brown JK, Nio-Kobayashi J, Abidin HBZ, Adin ZEHA, Boswell L, Burgess S, Lee K-F, Duncan WC (2014) The association between smoking and ectopic pregnancy: why nicotine is BAD for your fallopian tube. PLOS ONE 9, 2. www.plosone.org/article/info%3Adoi%2F10.1371%2Fjournal.pone.0089400, accessed 18 June 2014.
14. Narvekar SA, Gupta N, Shetty N, Kottur A, Srinivas M and Rao KA (2010) Does local endometrial injury in the nontransfer cycle improve the IVF-ET outcome in the subsequent cycle in patients with previous unsuccessful IVF? A randomized controlled pilot study. *J Hum Reprod Sci 3*, 1: 15–19.
15. Ma SX, Yin DE and Zhu YL (2005) Clinical observation on effect of Chinese herbs in adjusting hypoestrogenemia status by clomiphene to promote ovulation. *Zhongguo Zhong Xi Yi Jie He Za Zhi 25*, 4: 360–362.
16. Diamanti-Kandarakis E, Kandarakis H and Legro RS (2006) The role of genes and environment in the etiology of PCOS. *Endocrine 30*, 1: 19–26.
17. Burcelin R, Thorens B, Glauser M, Gaillard RC and Pralong FP (2003) Gonadotropin-releasing hormone secretion from hypothalamic neurons: stimulation by insulin and potentiation by leptin. *Endocrinology 144*, 10: 4484–4491.
18. Storlien LH, Jenkins AB, Chisholm DJ, Pacoe WS, Khouri S and Kraegen EW (1991) Influence of dietary fat composition on development of insulin resistance in rats. Relationship to muscle triglyceride and omega-3 fatty acids in muscle phospholid. *Diabetes 40*, 2: 280–289.
19. Lovejoy J and DiGirolamo M (1992) Habitual dietary intake and insulin sensitivity in lean and obese adults. *American Journal of Clinical Nutrition 55*, 6: 1174–1179.
20. Lim CE and Wong WS (2010) Current evidence of acupuncture on polycystic ovarian syndrome. *Gynecological Endocrinology 26*, 6: 473–478.
21. Jedel E, Labrie F, Odén A, Holm G, *et al.* (2011) Impact of electro-acupuncture and physical exercise on hyperandrogenism and oligo/amenorrhea in women with polycystic ovary syndrome: a randomized controlled trial. *American Journal of Physiology – Endocrinology and Metabolism 300*, 1: E37–E45.
22. Zhang J, Li T, Zhou L, Tang L, Xu L, Wu T, Lim DCE *et al.* (2010) Chinese herbal medicine for subfertile women with polycystic ovarian syndrome (Review); The Cochrane Collaboration. www.update-software.com/BCP/WileyPDF/EN/CD007535.pdf, accessed 30 July 2014.
23. Wild S, Roglic G, Green A, Sicree R and King H (2004) Global prevalence of diabetes. *Diabetes Care 27*: 1047–1053.
24. Goglia F (2005) Biological effects of 3,5-Diiodothyronine (T_2). *Biochemistry* (Moscow) *70*, 2: 164–172. Translated from *Biokhimiya 70*, 2: 203–213.
25. Poongothai S and Balasubramanian J (2012) A criticism on biological concepts of diiodothyronine. *Discovery Proteins 1*, 1: 22–26.
26. Schmidt PJ, Grover GN, Roy-Byrne PP and Rubinow DR (1993) Thyroid function in women with premenstrual syndrome. *J Clin Endocrinol Metab 76*, 3: 671–674.
27. Kaipia A and Hsueh AJ (1997) Regulation of ovarian follicle atresia. *Annu Rev Physiol 59*: 349–63.
28. Jiang JY, Cheung CK, Wang Y and Tsang BK (2003) Regulation of cell death and cell survival gene expression during ovarian follicular development and atresia. *Front Biosci 8*: 222–237.
29. Visser JA, de Jong FH, Joop Laven JSE and Themmen APN (2006) Anti-Müllerian hormone: a new marker for ovarian function Reproduction 6: 131 1–1319.
30. Kevenaar ME, Meerasahib MF, Kramer P, van de Lang-Born BMN, de Jong FH, Groome NP, Themmen APN and Visser JA (2006). Serum anti-Müllerian hormone levels reflect the size of the primordial follicle pool in mice. *Endocrinology 147*, 76: 3228–3234.
31. Gougeon A, Echochard R and Thalabard JC (1994) Age-related changes of the population of human ovarian follicles: increase in the disappearance rate of non-growing and early-growing follicles in aging women. *Biol Reprod 50*, 3: 653–63.

32. Murray A, Bennett CE, Perry JRB, Weedon MN, *et al.* (2011) Common genetic variants are significant risk factors for early menopause: results from the Breakthrough Generations Study. *Hum Mol Genet 20*, 1: 186–192.

Chapter 6

1. Developing Patient Partnerships (2006) Stress and Wellbeing 2006. www.unionsafety.eu/pdf_files/DPPStressAndWellbeingReport.pdf, accessed 17 May 2014.
2. Barrow B (2011) 'Stress "is top cause of workplace sickness" and is so widespread it's dubbed the "Black Death of the 21st century"'. *Daily Mail*, 5 October. www.dailymail.co.uk/health/article-2045309/Stress-Top-cause-workplace-sickness-dubbed-Black-Death-21st-century.html, accessed 10 June 2014.
3. Health and Safety Executive (2013) Stress and Psychological Disorders in Great Britain 2013. www.hse.gov.uk/statistics/causdis/stress/stress.pdf, accessed 30 July 2014.
4. Health and Safety Executive (2013) Stress and psychosocial disorders in Great Britain 2013. www.hse.gov.uk/statistics, accessed 17 May 2014.
5. Turcotte M (2011) Women and Health, Women in Canada: A gender-based statistical report. www.statcan.gc.ca/pub/89-503-x/2010001/article/11543-eng.pdf, accessed 30 July 2014.
6. Clay RA (2011) Stressed in America. American Psychological Association 42, 1. www.apa.org/monitor/2011/01/stressed-america.aspx, accessed 4 November 2013.
7. Russ T, Stamatakis E, Hamer M, Starr J, Kivmaki M and Batty G. (2012) Association between psychological distress and mortality: individual participant pooled analysis of 10 prospective cohort studies. *BMJ 345*: e4933.
8. Aldwin CM, Molitor N-T, Spiro A, Levenson MR, Molitor J and Igarashi H (2011) Do stress trajectories predict mortality in older men? Longitudinal findings from the VA Normative Aging Study. *Journal of Aging Research*. http://dx.doi.org/10.4061/2011/896109. accessed 30 July 2014.
9. Finegold JA, Asaria P and Francis DP (2012) Mortality from ischaemic heart disease by country, region, and age: statistics from World Health Organization and United Nations. *International Journal of Cardiology 168*, 2: 934–945.
10. Novak M, Björck L, Giang KW, Heden-Ståhl C, Wilhelmsen L and Rosengren A (2013) Perceived stress and incidence of type 2 diabetes: a 35-year follow-up study of middle-aged Swedish men. *Diabetic Medicine 30*, 1: e8–e16.
11. Szabo S, Tache Y and Somgyi A (2012) The legacy of Hans Selye and the origins of stress research: A retrospective 75 years after his landmark brief "Letter" to the Editor of Nature. *Stress 15*, 5: 472–478.
12. Lupien SJ, Maheu F, Tu M, Fiocco A and Schramek TE (2007) The effects of stress and stress hormones on human cognition: implications for the field of brain and cognition. *Brain and Cognition 65*, 3: 209–237.
13. Lupien SJ, Maheu F, Tu M, Fiocco A and Schramek TE (2007) The effects of stress and stress hormones on human cognition: implications for the field of brain and cognition. *Brain and Cognition 65*, 3: 209–237.
14. Bosma H, Marmot MG, Hemingway H, Nicholson AC, Brunner E and Stansfeld SA (1997) Low job control and risk of coronary heart disease in Whitehall II (prospective cohort) study. *BMJ 314*, 7080: 558–565.
15. Kuper H and Marmot M (2003) Job strain, job demands, decision latitude, and risk of coronary heart disease within the Whitehall II study. *J Epidemiol Community Health 57*: 147–153, doi: 10.1136/jech.57.2.147.
16. Ferrie JE (ed.) (2004) *Work Stress and Health: The Whitehall II Study*. London: Cabinet Office. www.ucl.ac.uk/whitehallII/pdf/Whitehallbooklet_1_.pdf, accessed 17 February 2014.
17. Möller-Leimkühler AM (2002) Barriers to help-seeking by men: a review of sociocultural and clinical literature with particular reference to depression. *Journal of Affective Disorders 71*, 1–3: 1–9.
18. Taylor SE, Klein LC, Lewis BP, Gruenewald TL, Gurung RAR and Updegraff JA (2000) Biobehavioral responses to stress in females: tend-and-befriend, not fight-or-flight. *Psychological Review 107*, 3: 411–429. Cited in Azar B (2000) A new stress paradigm for women. *American Psychological Association 31*, 7: 42.

19. Nolen-Hoeksema S, Larson J and Grayson C (1999) Explaining the gender difference in depressive symptoms. *Journal of Personality and Social Psychology 77*, 5: 1061–1072.
20. Taylor SE, Klein LC, Lewis BP, Gruenewald TL, Gurung RAR and Updegraff JA (2000) Biobehavioral responses to stress in females: tend-and-befriend, not fight-or-flight. *Psychological Review 107*, 3: 411–429. Cited in Azar B (2000) A new stress paradigm for women. *American Psychological Association 31*, 7: 42
21. Turcotte M (2011) Women and Health, Women in Canada: A gender-based statistical report. www.statcan.gc.ca/pub/89-503-x/2010001/article/11543-eng.pdf, accessed 30 July 2014.
22. Wang HX, Leineweber C, Kirkeeide R, Svane B, *et al.* (2007) Psychosocial stress and atherosclerosis: family and work stress accelerate progression of coronary disease in women. The Stockholm Female Coronary Angiography Study. *J Intern Med 261*, 3: 245–254.
23. Facchinetti F, Volpe A, Matteo ML, Genazzani AR and Artini GP (1997) An increased vulnerability to stress is associated with a poor outcome of in vitro fertilization-embryo transfer treatment. *Fert & Stert 67*, 2: 309–314.
24. Mauri C and Bosma A (2012) Immune regulatory function of B cells. *Annual Review of Immunology 30*: 221–241.
25. Vogelzangs N, Beekman ATF, Milaneschi Y, Bandinelli S, Ferrucci L and Penninx BWJH (2010) Urinary cortisol and six-year risk of all-cause and cardiovascular mortality. *J Clin Endocrinol Metab 95*, 11: 4959–4964.
26. Houck JC, Sharma VK, Patel YM and Gladner JA (1968) Induction of collagenolytic and proteolytic activities by anti-inflammatory drugs in the skin and fibroblast. *Biochem Pharmacol 17*, 10: 2081–2090.
27. Ebbesen SMS, Zachariae R, Mehlsen MY, Thomsen D, *et al.* (2009) Stressful life events are associated with a poor in-vitro fertilization (IVF) outcome: a prospective study. *Hum Reprod 24*, 9: 2173–2182.
28. Farrell K and Antoni MH (2010) Insulin resistance, obesity, inflammation, and depression in polycystic ovary syndrome: biobehavioral mechanisms and interventions. *Fert & Stert 94*, 5: 1565–1574.
29. Newcomer JW, Selke G, Melson AK, Gross J, Vogler GP and Dagogo-Jack S (1998) Dose-dependent cortisol-induced increases in plasma leptin concentration in healthy humans. *Arch Gen Psychiatry 55*, 11: 995–1000.
30. Wilcox G (2005) Insulin and insulin resistance. *Clin Biochem Rev 26*, 2: 19–39.
31. Nepomnaschy PA, Welch KB, McConnell DS, Low BS, Strassmann BI and England BG (2006) Cortisol levels and very early pregnancy loss in humans. *Proc Natl Acad Sci USA 103*, 10: 3938–3942.
32. Berger A (1999) Ritalin may influence serotonin balance in hyperactive children. *BMJ 318*, 212: 3.
33. Goodwin FK and Bunney WE Jr (1971) Depressions following reserpine: a reevaluation. *Semin Psychiatry 3*, 4: 435–448. Cited in Blier P (2001) Crosstalk between the norepinephrine and serotonin systems and its role in the antidepressant response. *J Psychiatry Neurosci 26* (Suppl.): S3–10.
34. Ben-Jonathan N and Hnasko R (2001) Dopamine as a prolactin (PRL) inhibitor. *Endocrine Reviews 22*, 6: 724–763.
35. Cosentino M, Rasini E, Colombo C, Marino F, et al. (2004) Dopaminergic modulation of oxidative stress and apoptosis in human peripheral blood lymphocytes: evidence for a D1-like receptor-dependent protective effect. *Free Radic Biol Med 36*, 10: 1233–1240.
36. Navarro-Beltran E (1999) Diccionario terminologico de ciencias medicas. Barcelona: Masson, p 91. Cited in Duque-Parra J (2005) Note on the Origin and History of the Term 'Apoptosis'. *The Anatomical Record 283*, B: 2–4.
37. Barlow Pugh M (ed.) (2000) *Stedman's Medical Dictionary.* Baltimore, MD: Lippincott Williams and Wilkins, p.113. Cited in Duque-Parra J 2005 Duque-Parra J; Note on the Origin and History of the Term "Apoptosis"; 2005; The Anatomical Record; (Part B: New Anat.) 283B:2-4
38. Oppenheim RW (1999) Programmed cell death. In Zigmond MJ, Bloom FE, Lan dis SC, Roberts JL and Squire LR (eds) *Fundamental neuroscience.* San Diego, CA: Academic Press, pp.581–609. Cited in Duque-Parra J (2005) Note on the Origin and History of the Term 'Apoptosis'. *The Anatomical Record 283*, B: 2–4.
39. Mattson MP (2000) Apoptosis in neurode-generative disorders. *Nat Rev Mol Cell Biol 1*: 120–129. Cited in Duque-Parra J (2005) Note on the Origin and History of the Term 'Apoptosis'. *The Anatomical Record 283*, B: 2–4.

40. Üstün TB, Ayuso-Mateos JL, Chatterji MH, Mathers C and Murray CJL (2004) Global burden of depressive disorders in the year 2000. *British Journal of Psychiatry 184*: 386–392.
41. Ferrari AJ, Charlson FJ, Norman RE, Patten SB, Freedman G, Murray CJL, Vos T and Whiteford HA (2013) Burden of depressive disorders by country, sex, age, and year: findings from the Global Burden of Disease Study 2010. *PLOS Medicine* (5 November). doi: 10.1371/journal.pmed.1001547.
42. Agarwal A, Saleh RA and Bedaiwy MA (2003) Role of reactive oxygen species in the pathophysiology of human reproduction. Fertility and Sterility 79, 4: 829–843.
43. Harvey AJ, Kind KL and Thompson JG (2002) REDOX regulation of early embryo development. *Reproduction 123*: 479–486.
44. Guerin P, El Mouatassim S and Menezo Y (2001) Oxidative stress and protection against reactive oxygen species in the preimplantation embryo and its surroundings. *Human Reprod Update 7*, 2: 175–189.
45. Agarwal A, Aponte-Mellado A, Premkumar BJ, Shaman A and Gupta S (2012) The effects of oxidative stress on female reproduction: a review. *Reproductive Biology and Endocrinology 10*: 49.

Chapter 7

1. Kessler RC, Berglund P, Demler O, Jin R, Merikangas KR and Walters EE (2005) Lifetime prevalence and age-of-onset distributions of DSM-IV disorders in the National Comorbidity Survey Replication. *Arch Gen Psychiatry 62*: 593–602.
2. Centers for Disease Control and Prevention (2009) *National Health and Nutrition Examination Survey Data*. Hyattsville, MD: National Center for Health Statistics.
3. Adam TC, Hasson RE, Ventura EE, Toledo-Corral C, *et al.* (2010) Cortisol is negatively associated with insulin sensitivity in overweight Latino youth. *J Clin Endocrinol Metab 95*, 10: 4729–4735.
4. Epel ES, McEwen B, Seeman T, Matthews K, *et al.* (2000) Stress and body shape: stress-induced cortisol secretion is consistently greater among women with central fat. *Psychosomatic Medicine 62*, 5: 623–632.
5. Babyak M, Blumenthal JA, Herman S, Khatri P, *et al.* (2000) Exercise treatment for major depression: maintenance of therapeutic benefit at 10 months. *Psychosom Med 62*, 5: 633–638.
6. Dunn AL, Trivedi MH, Kampert JB, Clark CG and Chambliss HO (2005) Exercise treatment for depression: efficacy and dose response. *American Journal of Preventive Medicine 28*, 1: 1–8.
7. Petruzzello SJ, Landers DM, Hatfield BD, Kubitz KA and Salazar W (1991) A meta-analysis on the anxiety-reducing effects of acute and chronic exercise. Outcomes and mechanisms. *Sports Medicine 11*, 3: 143–182.
8. Otis CL, Drinkwater B, Johnson M, Loucks A and Wilmore J (1997) American College of Sports Medicine position stand. The Female Athlete Triad. *Medicine and Science in Sports and Exercise 29*, 5: i–ix.
9. Female Athlete Triad Coalition (2014) For Professionals. www.femaleathletetriad.org/for-professionals/ and Position Stands, www.femaleathletetriad.org/for-professionals/position-stands, accessed 11 Jun 2014.
10. Cahill LE, Chiuve SE, Mekary RA, Jensen MK, Flint AJ, Hu FB and Rimm EB (2013) Prospective study of breakfast eating and incident coronary heart disease in a cohort of male US health professionals. *Circulation 128*: 337–343.
11. Maciocia G (1989) *The Foundations of Chinese Medicine: A Comprehensive Text for Acupuncturists and Herbalists*. Edinburgh: Churchill Livingstone.
12. Lyttleton J (2004) *Treatment of Infertility with Chinese Medicine*. Edinburgh: Churchill Livingstone.
13. Sakata K, Matumura Y, Yoshimura N, Tamaki J, Hashimoto T, Oguri S, Okayama A and Yanagawa H (2001) Relationship between skipping breakfast and cardiovascular disease risk factors in the national nutrition survey data. *Japanese Journal of Public Health 48*, 10: 837–884.
14. Boden G, Ruiz J, Urbain JL and Chen X (1996) Evidence for a circadian rhythm of insulin secretion. *Am J Physiol 271*, 2 Pt 1: E246–252.
15. Science Daily (2003) Night work may impair glucose tolerance. www.sciencedaily.com/releases/2013/06/130603114146.htm, accessed on 21 November 2013.

16. Pan A, Schernhammer ES, Sun Q and Hu FB (2011) Rotating night shift work and risk of type 2 diabetes: two prospective cohort studies in women. *Plos Medicine*, doi: 10.1371/journal.pmed.1001141.
17. Central Intelligence Agency (2013) The world factbook. www.cia.gov/library/publications/the-world-factbook, accessed 21 November 2013.

Chapter 8

1. van Haaften R, Haenen G, Evelo C and Bast A (2003) Effect of vitamin E on glutathione-dependent enzymes. *DMR 35*, 2–3: 215–253.
2. Yanardag R, Ozsoy-Sacan O, Ozdil S and Bolkent S (2007) Combined effects of vitamin C, vitamin E, and sodium selenate supplementation on absolute ethanol-induced injury in various organs of rats. *Int J Toxico 26*, 6: 513–523.
3. Sies H, Stahl W and Sevanian A (2005) Nutritional, dietary and postprandial oxidative stress. *Nutr 135*, 5: 969–972.
4. Linster CL and Van Schaftingen E (2007) Vitamin C. Biosynthesis, recycling and degradation in mammals. *FEBS J 274*, 1: 1–22.
5. Patrick L (2002) Mercury toxicity and antioxidants: Part 1: role of glutathione and alpha-lipoic acid in the treatment of mercury toxicity. *Alt Med Rev 7*, 6: 456–471.
6. Kumar C, Igbaria AD, Autreaux B, Planson AG, *et al.* (2011) Glutathione revisited: a vital function in iron metabolism and ancillary role in thiol-redox control. *EMBO Journal 30*, 10: 2044–2056.
7. Henshel D (2004) Control of glutathione synthesis in early embryo development. *Toxicol Sci 81*, 2: 257–259.
8. Trocino RA, Akazawa S, Ishibashi M, Matsumoto K, *et al.* (1995) Significance of glutathione depletion and oxidative stress in early embryogenesis in glucose-induced rat embryo culture. *Diabetes 44*, 8: 992–998.
9. Zhang D, Luo WY, Liao H, Wang CF and Sun Y (2008) The effects of oxidative stress to PCOS. *Sichuan Da Xue Xue Bao Yi Xue Ban 39*, 3: 421–423.
10. Phelan N, O'Connor A, Kyaw-Tun T, Correia N, Boran G, Roche HM and Gibney J (2010) Lipoprotein subclass patterns in women with polycystic ovary syndrome (PCOS) compared with equally insulin-resistant women without PCOS. J Clin Endocrinol Metab 95, 8: 3933–3999.
11. Henmi H, Endo T, Kitajima Y, Manase K, Hata H and Kudo R (2003) Effects of ascorbic acid supplementation on serum progesterone levels in patients with a luteal phase defect. *Fertil Steril 80*, 2: 459–461.
12. Kivity S, Agmon-Levin N, Zisappl M, Shapira Y, Nagy EV, Dankó K, Szekanecz Z, Langevitz P and Shoenfeld Y (2011) Vitamin D and autoimmune thyroid diseases. *Cellular & Molecular Immunology 8*: 243–248.
13. Ip C and Lisk DJ (1994) Bioactivity of selenium from Brazil nut for cancer prevention and selenoenzyme maintenance. *Nutr Cancer 21*, 3: 203–212.
14. Rodgers RJ, Lavranos TC, Rodgers HF, Young FM and Vella CA (1995) The physiology of the ovary: maturation of ovarian granulosa cells and a novel role for antioxidants in the corpus luteum. *J Steroid Biochem Mol Biol 53*: 241–246.
15. Krammer G and Aurich J (2010) Effect of intramuscularly administered beta-carotene on reproductive performance in sows. *Berl Munch Tierarztl Wochenschr 123*, 11–12: 496–499.
16. Brief S and Chew BP (1985) Effects of vitamin A and beta-carotene on reproductive performance in gilts. *J Anim Sci. 60*, 4: 998–1004.
17. Kamenova P (2006) Improvement of insulin sensitivity in patients with type 2 diabetes mellitus after oral administration of alpha-lipoic acid. *Hormones (Athens) 5*, 4: 251–258.
18. van Blerkom J (1998) Epigenetic influences on oocyte developmental competence: perifollicular vascularity and intrafollicular oxygen. *J Assist Reprod Genet 15*, 5: 226–234.
19. US National Library of Medicine (2014) Pthalates. http://toxtown.nlm.nih.gov/text_version/chemicals.php?id=24, accessed 18 May 2014.
20. McLachlan JA, Simpson E and Martin M (2006) Endocrine disrupters and female reproductive health. *Best Pract Res Clin Endocrinol Metab 20*, 1: 63–75.
21. Nicolopoulou-Stamati P and Pitsos MA (2001) The impact of endocrine disrupters on the female reproductive system. *Human Reproduction Update 7*, 3: 323–330.

22. Petro EM, Leroy JL, Covaci A, Fransen E, *et al.* (2012) Endocrine-disrupting chemicals in human follicular fluid impair in vitro oocyte developmental competence. *Hum Reprod 27*, 4: 1025–1033.
23. Diamanti-Kandarakis E, Bourguignon J-P, Giudice LC, Hauser R, *et al.* (2009) Endocrine-disrupting chemicals: an Endocrine Society scientific statement. *Endocrine Reviews 30*, 4: 293–342.
24. Eisenberg ML, Li S, Behr B, Cullen MR, Galusha D, Lamb DJ and Lipshultz LI (2014) Semen quality, infertility and mortality in the USA. *Hum Reprod.* doi: 10.1093/humrep/deu106.
25. Carlsen E, Giwercman A, Keiding N and Skakkebaek NE (1992) Evidence for decreasing quality of semen during past 50 years. *BMJ 305*, 6854:.609–613.
26. Rogers L (2012) Male infertility is soaring. So why do doctors keep blaming the woman when she can't have a baby? FEMAIL investigates. *Mail Online* (5 December). www.dailymail.co.uk/femail/article-2243642/Male-infertility-soaring-So-doctors-blaming-woman-baby-FEMAIL-investigates.html, accessed 5 June 2014.
27. *Time Magazine* (1984) Medicine: the saddest epidemic (10 September). http://content.time.com/time/magazine/article/0,9171,952515,00.html, accessed 5 June 2014.
28. Jensen TK, Sobotka T, Hansen MA, Pedersen AT, Lutz W and Skakkebæk NE (2008) Declining trends in conception rates in recent birth cohorts of native Danish women: a possible role of deteriorating male reproductive health. *International Journal of Andrology 31*, 2: 81–92.
29. Joffe M (2010) What has happened to human fertility? *Hum Reprod 25*, 2: 295–307.
30. Andersson AM, Jørgensen N, Main KM, Toppari J, Rajpert-De Meyts E, Leffers H, Juul A, Jensen TK and Skakkebæk NE (2008) Adverse trends in male reproductive health: we may have reached a crucial 'tipping point'. *International Journal of Andrology 31*, 2: 74–80.
31. Huyghe E, Matsuda T and Thonneau P (2003) Increasing incidence of testicular cancer worldwide: a review. *Journal of Urology 170*, 1: 5–11.
32. Garner MJ, Turner MC, Ghadirian P and Krewski D (2005) Epidemiology of testicular cancer: An overview. *International Journal of Cancer 116*, 3: 331–339.
33. Jensen TK, Jacobsen R, Christensen K, Nielsen NC and Bostofte E (2009) Good semen quality and life expectancy: a cohort study of 43,277 men. *American Journal of Epidemiology 170*, 5: 559–565.
34. Rolland M, Le Moal J, Wagner V, Royère D and De Mouzonl J (2013) Decline in semen concentration and morphology in a sample of 26,609 men close to general population between 1989 and 2005 in France. *Hum Reprod 28*, 2: 462–470.
35. Belyaev DK (1969) Domestication of animals. *Science Journal (UK) 5*: 24–29, 60–64. Cited in Trut L (1999) Early canid domestication: the farm-fox experiment. *Am Scientist 87*: 160–169.
36. Belyaev DK and Trut, LN (1982) Accelerating evolution. *Science in the USSR 5*: 24–29, 60–64. Cited in Trut L (1999) Early canid domestication: the farm-fox experiment. *Am Scientist 87*: 160–169.
37. Savolainen P, Zhang Y, Luo J, Lundeberg J and Leitner T (2002) Genetic evidence for an East Asian origin of domestic dogs. *Science 298*: 1610–1613.
38. Huxley J. Evolution: *The Modern Synthesis.* Cambridge, MA: MIT Press.
39. de Boo HA and Harding JE. The developmental origins of adult disease (Barker) hypothesis. *Australian and New Zealand Journal of Obstetrics and Gynaecology 46*: 4–14.
40. Banning C (1946) Food shortage and public health, first half of 1945. Special issue: The Netherlands during German Occupation. *Annals of the American Academy of Political and Social Science 245*, 93–110.
41. Roseboома TJ, van der Meulena JHP, Osmonde C, Barkere DJP, *et al.* Coronary heart disease after prenatal exposure to the Dutch famine, 1944–45. *Heart 84*: 595–598.
42. Elias S, Peeters P, Grobbee D and van Noord P (2004) Breast cancer risk after caloric restriction during the 1944–1945 Dutch famine. *J Natl Cancer Inst 96*: 539–546. Cited in Bromfeld J, Messamore W and Albertini D (2007) Epigenetic regulation during mammalian oogenesis. *Reproduction, Fertility and Development 20*, 95–6: 5–6.
43. Elias S, Peeters P, Grobbee D and van Noord P (2004) The 1944–1945 Dutch famine and subsequent overall cancer incidence. *Cancer Epidemiol Biomarkers Prev 14*: 1981–1985. Cited in Bromfeld J, Messamore W and Albertini D (2007) Epigenetic regulation during mammalian oogenesis. *Reproduction, Fertility and Development 20*, 95–6: 5–6.

44. Elias S, van Noord P, Peeters P, den Tonkelaar I and Grobbee D (2005) Childhood exposure to the 1944–1945 Dutch famine and subsequent female reproductive function. *Hum Reprod 20*: 2483–2488. Cited in Bromfeld J, Messamore W and Albertini D (2007) Epigenetic regulation during mammalian oogenesis. *Reproduction, Fertility and Development 20*, 95–6: 5–6.
45. Roseboom T, van der Meulen J, Ravelli A, Osmond C, Barker D, Bleker O (2001) Effects of prenatal exposure to the Dutch famine on adult disease in later life: an overview. *Mol Cell Endocrinol 185*: 93–98. Cited in Bromfeld J, Messamore W and Albertini D (2007) Epigenetic regulation during mammalian oogenesis. *Reproduction, Fertility and Development 20*, 95–6: 5–6.
46. Cropley JE, Suter CM, Beckman KB and Marti DIK (2006) Germ-line epigenetic modification of the murine A^{vy} allele by nutritional supplementation. *PNAS 103*, 46: 17308–17312.
47. de Boo HA and Harding JE (2006) The developmental origins of adult disease (Barker) hypothesis. *Australian and New Zealand Journal of Obstetrics and Gynaecology 46*, 1: 4–14.
48. Reik W, Dean W and Walter J. (2006) Epigenetic reprogramming in mammalian development. *Science 293*: 1089–1093. Cited in de Boo HA and Harding JE (2006) The developmental origins of adult disease (Barker) hypothesis. *Australian and New Zealand Journal of Obstetrics and Gynaecology 46*, 1: 4–14.

Chapter 9

1. Cochrane AL (1972) *Effectiveness and Efficiency: Random Reflections on Health Services*. London: Nuffield Provincial Hospitals Trust, p.31. Cited in http://en.wikipedia.org, Placebo.
2. Saunders W (2004) Halloween and All Saints Day. CatholicCulture.org. www.catholicculture.org/culture/library/view.cfm?recnum=6210, accessed 21 February 2014.
3. Online Etymology Dictionary. www.etymonline.com, accessed 2 December 2013.
4. Motherby G (1785) A New Medical Dictionary (2nd edn). Cited in de Craen AJM, Kaptchuk TJ, Tijssen JGP and Kleijnen J (1999) Placebos and placebo effects in medicine: historical overview. *J R Soc Med 92*: 511–515.
5. House of Commons Science and Technology Committee (2010) Evidence Check 2; Homeopathy, HC45. London: TSO.
6. Kaiser HE Bodey B Jr, Siegel SE, Gröger AM, Bodey B (2000) Spontaneous neoplastic regression: the significance of apoptosis. *In Vivo 14*, 6: 773–788.
7. Del Giudice I, Chiaretti S, Tavolaro S, De Propris M, et al. (2009) Spontaneous regression of chronic lymphocytic leukemia: Clinical and biologic features of 9 cases. *Blood 114*, 3: 638–646.
8. Everson TC, Cole WH (1968) *Spontaneous Regression of Cancer.* Philadelphia, PA: JB Saunders, p.4.
9. Papac RJ (1998) Spontaneous regression of cancer: Possible mechanisms. *In Vivo 12*, 6: 571–578.
10. Hobohm U (2001) Fever and cancer in perspective. *Cancer Immunol Immunother 50*, 8: 391–396. Cited in McCarthy E (2006) The toxins of William B Coley and the treatment of bone and soft tissue sarcomas. *Iowa Orthop J 26*: 154–158.
11. Kleef R, Jonas WB, Knogler W and Stenzinger W (2001) Fever, cancer incidence and spontaneous remissions. *Neuroimmunomodulation 9*, 2: 55–64.
12. Richardson MA, Ramirez T, Russell NC and Moye LA (1999) Coley toxins immunotherapy: a retrospective review. *Altern Ther Health Med 5*, 3: 42–47.
13. Jessy T (2011) Immunity over inability: the spontaneous regression of cancer. *J Nat Sci Biol Med 2*, 1: 43–49.
14. McQuay H, Carroll D and Moore A (1996) Variation in the placebo effect in randomised controlled trials of analgesics: all is as blind as it seems. *Pain 64*, 2: 331–335.
15. van Leeuwen JH, Castro R, Busse M and Bemelmans BL (2006) The placebo effect in the pharmacologic treatment of patients with lower urinary tract symptoms. *Eur Urol 50*, 3: 440–453.
16. Kienle GS and Kiene H (1996) Placebo effect and placebo concept: a critical methodological and conceptual analysis of reports on the magnitude of the placebo effect. *Alternative Therapies in Health and Medicine 2*, 6: 39–54.
17. Flaten MA, Simonsen T and Olsen H (1999) Drug-related information generates placebo and nocebo responses that modify the drug response. *Psychosom Med 61*, 2: 250–255.

18. Maruta T, Colligan RC, Malinchoc M and Offord KP (2000) Optimists vs pessimists: survival rate among medical patients over a 30-year period. *Mayo Clin Proc 75*, 2: 140–143. Cited in Mindfulness and positive thinking, www.pursuit-of-happiness.org/science-of-happiness/positive-thinking, accessed 1 December 2013.
19. Segerstrom SC and Sephton SE (2010) Optimistic expectancies and cell-mediated immunity: the role of positive affect, doi: 10.1177/0956797610362061. Cited in Mindfulness and positive thinking, www.pursuit-of-happiness.org/science-of-happiness/positive-thinking, accessed 1 December 2013.
20. Lancastle D and Boivin J (2005) Dispositional optimism, trait anxiety, and coping: unique or shared effects on biological response to fertility treatment? *Health Psychology 24*, 2: 171–178.
21. Kaptchuk TJ, Kelley JM and Lembo AJ (2008) Components of placebo effect: randomised controlled trial in patients with irritable bowel syndrome. *BMJ 336*, 7651: 999–1003.
22. Jarcho JM, Mayer EA and London ED (2009) Neuroimaging placebo effects: new tools generate new questions. *Clin Pharmacol Ther 86*, 4: 352–354.
23. Watson A, El-Deredy W, Iannetti GD, Lloyd D, *et al.* (2009) Placebo conditioning and placebo analgesia modulate a common brain network during pain anticipation and perception. *Pain 145*, 1–2: 24–30.
24. BMJ (2014) Clinical Evidence Efficacy Categorisations: What conclusions has *Clinical Evidence* drawn about what works, what doesn't based on randomised controlled trial evidence? http://clinicalevidence.bmj.com/x/set/static/cms/efficacy-categorisations.html accessed 19 May 2014.
25. Stener Victorin E, Waldenstrom U, Tagnfors U, Lundeberg T, Lindstedt G and Per Janson O (2000) Effects of electro-acupuncture on anovulation in women with polycystic ovary syndrome. *Acta Obstetricia et Gynecologica Scandinavica 79*, 3: 180–188.
26. Sackett DL, Rosenberg WM, Gray JA, Haynes RB and Richardson WS (1996) Evidence based medicine: what it is and what it isn't. *BMJ 312*, 7023: 71–72.
27. Sackett L, Gray M, Haynes B and Richardson S (1996) Evidenced based medicine: what it is and what it isn't. *BMJ 312*, 7023: 71–72.
28. Dobbie AE, Schneider FD, Anderson AD and Littlefield J (2000) What evidence supports teaching evidence-based medicine? *Acad Med 75*, 12: 1184–1185. Cited in Cohen AM, Stavri PZ and Hersh WR (2004) A categorization and analysis of the criticisms of evidence-based medicine. *International Journal of Medical Informatics 73*, 35–43.
29. Sehon SR and Stanley DE (2003) A philosophical analysis of the evidence-based medicine debate. *BMC Health Serv Res 3*, 1: 14. Cited in Cohen AM, Stavri PZ and Hersh WR (2004) A categorization and analysis of the criticisms of evidence-based medicine. *International Journal of Medical Informatics 73*, 35–43.
30. Bonisteel P (2009) The tyranny of evidence-based medicine. *Canadian Family Physician 55*, 10: 979.
31. Holmes D, Murray S, Perron A and Rail G (2006) Deconstructing the evidence-based discourse in health sciences: truth, power and fascism. *Int J Evid Based Health 4*: 180–186.
32. Mykhalovskey E and Weir L (2004) The problem of evidence-based medicine: directions for social science. *Social Science & Medicine 59*: 1059–1069, p.1062.
33. Jacobson L, Edwards A, Granier S and Butler C (1997) Evidence-based medicine and general practice. *British Journal of General Practice 47*: 449–452. Cited in Mykhalovskey E and Weir L (2004) The problem of evidence-based medicine: directions for social science. *Social Science and Medicine 59*: 1059–1069, p.1062.
34. Holmes D, Murray S, Perron A and Rail G (2006) Deconstructing the evidence-based discourse in health sciences: truth, power and fascism. *Int J Evid Based Health 4*: 180–186.
35. Holmes D, Murray S, Perron A and Rail G (2006) Deconstructing the evidence-based discourse in health sciences: truth, power and fascism. *Int J Evid Based Health 4*: 180–186.
36. Han J-S and Ho Y-S (2011) Global trends and performances of acupuncture research. *Neuroscience and Biobehavioral Reviews 35*: 680–687.
37. Paulus WE, Zhang M, Strehler E, Seybold B and Sterzik K (2003) Placebo-controlled trial of acupuncture effects in assisted reproduction therapy. The 19th Annual Meeting of the ESHRE, Xviii18.
38. So EW, Ng EH, Wong YY, Lau EY, Yeung WS and Ho PC (2009) A randomized double blind comparison of real and placebo acupuncture in IVF treatment. *Hum Reprod 24*, 2: 341–348.
39. Stener-Victorin E (2009) Acupuncture in in vitro fertilisation: why do reviews produce contradictory results? *Focus Altern Complement Ther 14*: 8–11.

40. Benedetti F (2014) Drugs and placebos: what's the difference? Understanding the molecular basis of the placebo effect could help clinicians to better use it in clinical practice. *EMBO Reports 15*, 4: 329–332.
41. Cited in J Macrum (2012) *The Virtuous Physician: The Role of Virtue in Medicine.* New York: Springer.
42. Landau RL (1996) ... And the least of these is empathy. Cited in Spiro HM, McCrea MG, Peschel CE and St James D (eds) *Empathy and the Practice of Medicine: Beyond Pills and the Scalpel.* New Haven, CT: Yale University Press.
43. MacLean PD (1967) The brain in relation to empathy and medical education. *Journal of Nervous and Mental Disease 144*, 5: 374–382. Cited in Racine E (2006) What role should emotions and empathy play in ethical decision making? *Canadian Psychiatry Aujourd'hui 2*, 6. http://publications.cpa-apc.org/browse/documents/121, accessed 30 July 2014.
44. BMJ (1952) The bottle of medicine. *British Medical Journal 1*: 149.
45. Larre C and Rochat de La Vallee E (1990) The practitioner–patient relationship: wisdom from the Chinese classics. *Journal of Traditional Acupuncture* (Winter): 14–17, p.14.
46. Spiegel D, Bloom JR, Kraemer HC, Gottheil E (1989) Effect of psychosocial treatment on survival of patients with metastatic breast cancer. *Lancet 2*, 8668: 888–891.
47. Spiegel D, Butler LD, Giese-Davis J, Koopman C, et al. (2007) Effects of supportive-expressive group therapy on survival of patients with metastatic breast cancer. *Cancer 110*, 5: 1130–1138.
48. Satin JR, Linden W, Phillips MJ (2009) Depression as a predictor of disease progression and mortality in cancer patients: a meta-analysis. *Cancer 115*, 2: 5349–5361.
49. Gallo JJ, Armenian HK, Ford DE, Eaton WW, Khachaturian AS (2000) Major depression and cancer: The 13-year follow-up of the Baltimore epidemiologic catchment area sample. *Cancer Causes and Control 11*, 8: 751–758.
50. Penninx BWJH, Guralnik JM, Havlik RJ (1998) Chronically Depressed Mood and Cancer Risk in Older Persons; *JNCI J Natl Cancer Inst 90*, 24: 1888–1893.
51. Kanesvaran R, Li H, Koo K-N, Poon D (2011) Analysis of Prognostic Factors of Comprehensive Geriatric Assessment and Development of a Clinical Scoring System in Elderly Asian Patients With Cancer. *JCO 29*, 27: 3620–3627.
52. Lamm C, Batson CD and Decety J (2007) The neural substrate of human empathy: effects of perspective-taking and cognitive appraisal. *Journal of Cognitive Science 19*, 1: 42–58.
53. Jensen KB, Petrovic P, Kerr CE, Kirsch I (2013) Sharing pain and relief: neural correlates of physicians during treatment of patients. *Molecular Psychiatry*, doi:10.1038/mp.2012.195.

Chapter 10

1. Verhaak CM, Smeenk JM, Evers AW, Kremer JA, Kraaimaat FW and Braat DD (2007) Women's emotional adjustment to IVF: a systematic review of 25 years of research. *Hum Reprod Update* 13, 1: 27–36.
2. Brandes M, van der Steen JO, Bokdam SB, Hamilton CJ *et al.* (2009) When and why do subfertile couples discontinue their fertility care? A longitudinal cohort study in a secondary care subfertility population. *Hum Reprod 24*, 12: 3127–3135.
3. Rajkhowa M, McConnell A and Thomas GE (2006) Reasons for discontinuation of IVF treatment: a questionnaire study. *Hum Reprod 21*, 2: 358–363.
4. Van den Broeck U, Holvoet L, Enzlin P, Bakelants E, Demyttenaere K and D'Hooghe T (2009) Reasons for dropout in infertility treatment. *Gynecol Obstet Invest 68*, 1: 58–64.
5. Verberg MF, Eijkemans MJ, Heijnen EM, Broekmans FJ, *et al.* (2008) Why do couples drop-out from IVF treatment? A prospective cohort study. *Hum Reprod 23*, 9: 2050–2055.
6. American Society for Reproductive Medicine (2014) Preparing for IVF: emotional considerations. www.asrm.org/detail.aspx?id=1902, accessed on 9 December 2013.
7. Mahlstedt PP, Macduff S and Bernstein J (1987) Emotional factors and the in vitro fertilization and embryo transfer process. *J In Vitro Fert Embryo Transf 4*, 4: 232–236.
8. National Institutes of Health, Office of Dietary Supplements (2013) Vitamin A: Fact sheet for consumers. http://ods.od.nih.gov/factsheets/VitaminA-Consumer, accessed 30 July 2014.
9. Stener-Victorin E, Waldenström U, Andersson SA and Wikland M (1996) Reduction of blood flow impedance in the uterine arteries of infertile women with electro-acupuncture. *Hum Reprod 11*, 6: 1314–1317.

10. Ho M, Huang L-C, Chang Y-Y, Chen H-Y, *et al.* (2009) Electroacupuncture reduces uterine artery blood flow impedance in infertile women. *Taiwanese Journal of Obstetrics and Gynecology 48*, 2: 148–151.
11. Thomas GD and Segal SS (2004) Neural control of muscle blood flow during exercise. *J Appl Physiol (1985) 97*, 2: 731–738.
12. Stener-Victorin E, Waldenstrom U, Nilsson L, Wikland M and Janson P (1999) A prospective randomized study of electro-acupuncture versus alfentanil as anaesthesia during oocyte aspiration in in-vitro fertilization. *Hum Reprod 14*: 2480–2484.
13. Stener-Victorin E, Waldenström U, Wikland M, Nilsson L, Hägglund L and Lundeberg T (2003) Electro-acupuncture as a peroperative analgesic method and its effects on implantation rate and neuropeptide Y concentrations in follicular fluid. *Hum Reprod 18*, 7: 1454–1460.
14. Sator-Katzenschlager SM, Wölfler MM, Kozek-Langenecker SA, Sator K, *et al.* (2006) Auricular electro-acupuncture as an additional perioperative analgesic method during oocyte aspiration in IVF treatment. *Hum Reprod 21*, 8: 2114–2120.
15. Paulus WE, Zhang M, Strehler E, El-Danasouri I, Sterzik K (2002) Influence of acupuncture on the pregnancy rate in patients who undergo assisted reproduction therapy. *Fertil Steril 77*, 4: 721–724.
16. Craig LB, Criniti AR, Hansen KR, Marshall LA and Soules MR (2007) Acupuncture lowers pregnancy rates when performed before and after embryo transfer. *Fertil Steril 88*. (Suppl 1): S40. (Abstract O–106). Cited in Manheimer E and Stener-Victorin E (2011) Commentary on the Cochrane Review of Acupuncture and Assisted Conception. *Explore (NY) 7*, 2: 120–123.
17. So EW, Ng EH, Wong YY, Lau EY, Yeung WS and Ho PC (2009) A randomized double blind comparison of real and placebo acupuncture in IVF treatment. *Hum Reprod 24*: 341–348. Cited in Manheimer E and Stener-Victorin E (2011) Commentary on the Cochrane Review of Acupuncture and Assisted Conception. *Explore (NY) 7*, 2: 120–123.
18. Paulus WE, Zhang M, Strehler E, Seybold B and Sterzik K (2003) Placebo-controlled trial of acupuncture effects in assisted reproduction therapy. The 19th Annual Meeting of the ESHRE, Xviii18.
19. de Lacey S and Smith C (2013) Acupuncture and infertility treatment: is there more to the outcome for women than pregnancy? *Medical Acupuncture 25*, 3: 195–199.
20. Khorram NM, Horton S, Sahakian V, Chacon R and Khorram O (2012) Adjuvant acupuncture reduces first trimester pregnancy loss after IVF. *OJOG 2*, 3: 283–286.
21. MacPherson H, Thorpe L, Thomas K and Geddes D (2004) Acupuncture for depression: first steps toward a clinical evaluation. *J Alt and Com Med 10*, 6: 1083–1091.
22. Smith CA, Hay PPJ, and MacPherson H (2010) Acupuncture for depression (Review). *Cochrane Database of Systematic Reviews 1*: 1–79. www.thecochranelibrary.com/userfiles/ccoch/file/Acupuncture_ancient_traditions/CD004046.pdf, accessed 30 July 2014.
23. Wang L, Sun DW, Zou W and Zhang JY (2008) Systematic evaluation of therapeutic effect and safety of acupuncture for treatment of depression. *Zhongguo Zhen Jiu 28*, 5: 381–386.
24. Wang H, Qi H, Wang B-S, Cui Y-Y, *et al.* (2008) Is acupuncture beneficial in depression: a meta-analysis of 8 randomized controlled trials? *Journal of Affective Disorders 111*, 2–3: 125–134.
25. Luo H, Meng F, Jia Y and Zhao X (1998) Clinical research on the therapeutic effect of the electro-acupuncture treatment in patients with depression. *Psychiatry and Clinical Neurosciences 52* (Suppl.): S338–S340.
26. Manber R, Schnyer RN, Allen JJB, Rush AJ and Blasey CM (2004) Acupuncture: a promising treatment for depression during pregnancy. *Journal of Affective Disorders 83*, 89–95.
27. Kim SYH and Holloway RG (2003) Burdens and benefits of placebo in antidepressant clinical trials: a decision and cost effectiveness analysis. *Am J Psychiatry 160*: 1272–1276. Cited in Manber R, Schnyer RN, Allen JJB, Rush AJ and Blasey CM (2004) Acupuncture: a promising treatment for depression during pregnancy. *Journal of Affective Disorders 83*, 89–95.
28. Yonkers KA, Dyck IR, Warshaw M and Keller MB (2000) Factors predicting the clinical course of generalised anxiety disorder. *Br J Psychitary 176*: 544–549. Cited in Arranz L, Guayerbas N, Siboni L and De la Fuente M (2007) Effect of acupuncture treatment on the immune function impairment found in anxious women. *American Journal of Chinese Medicine 35*, 1: 35–51.
29. Arranz L, Guayerbas N, Siboni L and De la Fuente M (2007) Effect of acupuncture treatment on the immune function impairment found in anxious women. *American Journal of Chinese Medicine 35*, 1: 35–51.

30. Víctor VM, Rocha M and De la Fuente M (2004) Immune cells: free radicals and antioxidants in sepsis. *Int Immunopharmacol 4*: 327–347. Cited in Arranz L, Guayerbas N, Siboni L and De la Fuente M (2007) Effect of acupuncture treatment on the immune function impairment found in anxious women. *American Journal of Chinese Medicine 35*, 1: 35–51.
31. Víctor VM, Rocha M and De la Fuente M (2003) Regulation of macrophage function by the antioxidant N-acetylcysteine in mouse-oxidative stress by endotoxin. *Int Immunopharmacol 3*: 97–106. Cited in Arranz L, Guayerbas N, Siboni L and De la Fuente M (2007) Effect of acupuncture treatment on the immune function impairment found in anxious women. *American Journal of Chinese Medicine 35*, 1: 35–51.
32. Smith JE, Richardson J, Hoffman C and Pilkington K (2005) Mindfulness-based stress reduction as supportive therapy in cancer care: systematic review. *Journal of Advanced Nursing 52*, 3: 315–327.
33. Irving JA, Dobkin PL and Park J (2009) Cultivating mindfulness in health care professionals: a review of empirical studies of mindfulness-based stress reduction (MBSR). *Complementary Therapies in Clinical Practice 15*: 61–66.
34. Toneatto T and Nguyen L (2007) Does mindfulness meditation improve anxiety and mood symptoms? A review of the controlled research. *Canadian Journal of Psychiatry/La Revue canadienne de psychiatrie 52*, 4: 260–266.
35. Sephton SE, Salmon P, Weissbecker I, Ulmer C, *et al.* (2007) Mindfulness meditation alleviates depressive symptoms in women with fibromyalgia: results of a randomized clinical trial. *Arthritis Rheum 57*, 1: 77–85.
36. Hofmann SG, Sawyer AT, Witt AA and Oh D (2010) The effect of mindfulness-based therapy on anxiety and depression: a meta-analytic review. *Journal of Consulting and Clinical Psychology 78*, 2: 169–183.
37. Reibel DK, Greeson JM, Brainard GC and Rosenzweig S (2001) Mindfulness-based stress reduction and health-related quality of life in a heterogeneous patient population. *General Hospital Psychiatry 23*, 4: 183–192.
38. Goldin PR and Gross JJ (2010) Effects of mindfulness-based stress reduction (MBSR) on emotion regulation in social anxiety disorder. *Emotion 10*, 1: 83–91.
39. Lavey R, Sherman T, Mueser KT, Osborne DD, Currier M and Wolfe R (2005) The effects of yoga on mood in psychiatric inpatients. *Psychiatric Rehabilitation Journal 28*, 4: 399–402, doi: 10.2975/28.2005.399.402.
40. Kuramoto AM (2006) Therapeutic benefits of Tai Chi exercise: research review. *Wisconsin Medical Journal 105*, 7: 42–46.
41. Kim SH, Kim YH, Kim HJ, Lee SH and Yu SO (2009) The effect of laughter therapy on depression, anxiety, and stress in patients with breast cancer undergoing radiotherapy. *J Korean Oncol Nurs 9*, 2: 155–162.
42. Bennett MP, Zeller JM, Rosenberg L and McCann J (2003) The effect of mirthful laughter on stress and natural killer cell activity. *Alternative Therapies in Health and Medicine 9*, 2: 38–45.
43. Nasir UM, Iwanaga S, Nabi AH, Urayama O, *et al.* (2005) Laughter therapy modulates the parameters of renin-angiotensin system in patients with type 2 diabetes. *Int J Molecular Medicine 16*, 6: 1077–1081.
44. Friedler S, Glasser S, Azani L, Freedman LS, *et al.* (2011) The effect of medical clowning on pregnancy rates after in vitro fertilization and embryo transfer. *Fert & Stert 95*, 6: 2127–2130.

Chapter 11

1. National Institutes of Health Office of Dietary Supplements (2013) Vitamin A: Fact sheet for consumers. http://ods.od.nih.gov/factsheets/VitaminA-QuickFacts, accessed 20 May 2014.
2. National Institutes of Health Office of Dietary Supplements (2011) Vitamin B6: Fact sheet for health professionals. http://ods.od.nih.gov/factsheets/VitaminB6-HealthProfessional, accessed 20 May 2014.
3. National Institutes of Health Office of Dietary Supplements (2013) Vitamin A: Fact sheet for consumers. http://ods.od.nih.gov/factsheets/VitaminA-QuickFacts, accessed 20 May 2014.
4. Pravst I, Zmitek K and Zmitek J (2010) Coenzyme Q10 contents in foods and fortification strategies. *Crit Rev Food Sci Nutr 50*, 4: 269–280.

5. University of Maryland Medical Center (2013) Coenzyme Q10; Complementary and Alternative Medicine Guide. https://umm.edu/health/medical/altmed/supplement/coenzyme-q10, accessed 30 July 2014.
6. National Institutes of Health Office of Dietary Supplements (2013) Vitamin C: Fact sheet for health professionals. http://ods.od.nih.gov/factsheets/VitaminC-HealthProfessional, accessed 20 May 2014.
7. Grajecki D, Zyriax BC and Buhling KJ (2012) The effect of micronutrient supplements on female fertility: a systematic review. *Archives of Gynecology and Obstetrics 285*, 5: 1463–1471.
8. Al-Katib SR, Al-Kaabi MMH and Al-Jashamy KA (2013) Effects of vitamin C on the endometrial thickness and ovarian hormones of progesterone and estrogen in married and unmarried women. *American Journal of Research Communication 1*, 8: 24–31.
9. Henmi H, Endo T, Kitajima Y, Manase K, Hata H and Kudo R. (2003) Effects of ascorbic acid supplementation on serum progesterone levels in patients with a luteal phase defect. *Fertil Steril 80*, 2: 459–461
10. Hathcock JN, Azzi A, Blumberg J, Bray T, *et al.* (2005) Vitamins E and C are safe across a broad range of intakes. *Am J Clin Nutr 81*: 736–745. Cited in Kucharski H and Zajac J (2009) *Handbook of Vitamin C Research: Daily Requirements, Dietary Sources and Adverse Effects.* Nutrition and Diet Research Progress Series. New York: Nova Science Publishers.
11. NHS Choices (2012) Vitamin D, Vitamins and Minerals: Vitamin D. www.nhs.uk/Conditions/vitamins-minerals/Pages/Vitamin-D.aspx, accessed 30 July 2014.
12. National Institutes of Health, Office of Dietary Supplements (2013) Vitamin E: Fact sheet for professionals. http://ods.od.nih.gov/factsheets/VitaminE-HealthProfessional, accessed 20 May 2014.
13. Brown BG, Zhao X-Q, Chait A, Fisher LD, Cheung MC, Morse JS, *et al.* (2001) Simvastatin and niacin, antioxidant vitamins, or the combination for the prevention of coronary disease. *N Engl J Med 345*: 1583–1592. Cited in National Institutes of Health Office of Dietary Supplements (2013) Vitamin E: Fact sheet for professionals. http://ods.od.nih.gov/factsheets/VitaminE-HealthProfessional, accessed 20 May 2014.
14. Cheung MC, Zhao X-Q, Chait A, Albers JJ and Brown BG (2001) Antioxidant supplements block the response of HDL to simvastatin-niacin therapy in patients with coronary artery disease and low HDL. *Arterioscler Thromb Vasc Biol 21*: 1320–1326. Cited in National Institutes of Health Office of Dietary Supplements (2013) Vitamin E: Fact sheet for professionals. http://ods.od.nih.gov/factsheets/VitaminE-HealthProfessional, accessed 20 May 2014.
15. Doyle C, Kushi LH, Byers T, Courneya KS, Demark-Wahnefried W, Grant B, et al., for the 2006 Nutrition, Physical Activity and Cancer Survivorship Advisory Committee (2006) Nutrition and physical activity during and after cancer treatment: an American Cancer Society guide for informed choices. *CA Cancer J Clin 56*: 323–353. Cited in National Institutes of Health Office of Dietary Supplements (2013) Vitamin E: Fact sheet for professionals. http://ods.od.nih.gov/factsheets/VitaminE-HealthProfessional, accessed 20 May 2014.
16. Lawenda BD, Kelly KM, Ladas EJ, Sagar SM, Vickers A and Blumberg JB (2008) Should supplemental antioxidant administration be avoided during chemotherapy and radiation therapy? *J Natl Cancer Inst 100*: 773–783. Cited in National Institutes of Health Office of Dietary Supplements (2013) Vitamin E: Fact sheet for professionals. http://ods.od.nih.gov/factsheets/VitaminE-HealthProfessional, accessed 20 May 2014.
17. Block KI, Koch AC, Mead MN, Tothy PK, Newman RA and Gyllenhaal C (2007) Impact of antioxidant supplementation on chemotherapeutic efficacy: a systematic review of the evidence from randomized controlled trials. *Cancer Treat Rev 33*: 407–418. Cited in National Institutes of Health Office of Dietary Supplements (2013) Vitamin E: Fact sheet for professionals. http://ods.od.nih.gov/factsheets/VitaminE-HealthProfessional, accessed 20 May 2014.
18. Geleijnse J, Vermeer C, Grobbee D, Schurgers L, *et al.* (2004) Dietary intake of menaquinone is associated with a reduced risk of coronary heart disease: The Rotterdam Study. *J. Nutr 134*, 11: 3100–3105.
19. Schurgers L, Spronk H, Soute B, Schiffers P, DeMey J, Vermeer C (2007) Regression of warfarin-induced medial elastocalcinosis by high intake of vitamin K in rats. *Blood 109*, 7: 2823–2931.
20. National Institutes of Health Clinical Center (2012) Important information to know when you are taking: Warfarin (Coumadin) and Vitamin K. www.cc.nih.gov/ccc/patient_education/drug_nutrient/coumadin1.pdf, accessed 16 June 2014.
21. Bates CJ (2009) *Vitamin K in Guide to Nutritional Supplements* (ed. B Caballero). Oxford: Elsevier, p.487.

22. National Institutes of Health Clinical Center, (2012) Important information to know when you are taking: Warfarin (Coumadin) and Vitamin K. www.cc.nih.gov/ccc/patient_education/drug_nutrient/coumadin1.pdf, accessed 16 June 2014.
23. Rhéaume-Bleue K (2012) *Vitamin K2 and the Calcium Paradox: How a Little-known Vitamin Could Save Your Life*. John Wiley & Sons Canada.
24. National Institutes of Health Office of Dietary Supplements (2013) Zinc: Fact sheet for health professionals. http://ods.od.nih.gov/factsheets/Zinc-HealthProfessional, accessed 16 June 2014.
25. Rebagliato M, Murcia M, Espada M, Alvarez-Pedrerol M, *et al.* (2010) Iodine intake and maternal thyroid function during pregnancy. *Epidemiology 21*, 1: 62–69. Cited in National Institutes for Health, Office of Dietary Supplements (2011) Iodine: Fact sheet for professionals. http://ods.od.nih.gov/factsheets/Iodine-HealthProfessional/#en3, accessed 30 July 2014.
26. NHS Choices (2012) Vitamins and minerals: Iodine. www.nhs.uk/Conditions/vitamins-minerals/Pages/Iodine.aspx, accessed 30 July 2014.
27. Teas J, Pino S, Critchley A and Braverman LE (2004) Variability of iodine content in common commercially available edible seaweeds. *Thyroid 14*, 10: 836–841.
28. Resnicow K (1991) The relationship between breakfast habits and plasma cholesterol levels in schoolchildren. *Journal of School Health 61*, 2: 81–85.
29. Berkey CS, Rockett HR, Gillman MW, Field AE and Colditz GA (2003) Longitudinal study of skipping breakfast and weight change in adolescents. *Int J Obes Relat Metab Disord 27*, 10: 1258–1266. Cited in Giovannini M, Verduci E, Scaglioni S, Salvatici E, *et al.* (2008) Breakfast: a good habit, not a repetitive custom. *Journal of International Medical Research* 36, 4: 613–624.
30. Utter J, Scragg R, Mhurchu CN and Schaaf D (2007) At-home breakfast consumption among New Zealand children: associations with body mass index and related nutrition behaviors. *J Am Diet Assoc 107*, 4: 570–576. Cited in Giovannini M, Verduci E, Scaglioni S, Salvatici E, *et al.* (2008) Breakfast: a good habit, not a repetitive custom. *Journal of International Medical Research* 36, 4: 613–624.
31. Ma Y, Bertone ER, Stanek EJ, Reed GW, *et al.* (2003) Association between eating patterns and obesity in a free-living US adult population. *Am J Epidemiol 158*, 1: 85–92.
32. Bazzano LA, Song Y, Bubes V, Good CK, Manson JE and Liu S (2005) Dietary intake of whole and refined grain breakfast cereals and weight gain in men. *Obesity Research 13*, 11: 1952–1960.
33. Cahill LE, Chiuve SE, Mekary RA, Jensen MK, *et al.* (2013) Prospective study of breakfast eating and incident coronary heart disease in a cohort of male US health professionals. *Circulation 128*: 337–343, doi: 10.1161/ CIRCULATIONAHA.113.001474.
34. Recipe kindly provided by George Cooper (2013) *Be Your Own Nutritionist: Rethink Your Relationship with Food*. London: Short Books.

INDEX

Note: page numbers in bold indicate major mentions